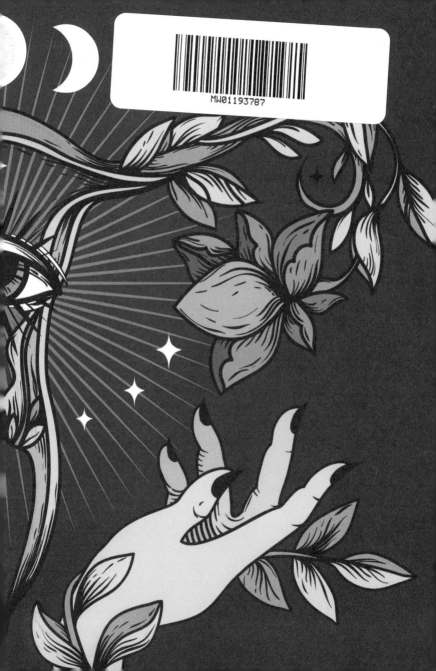

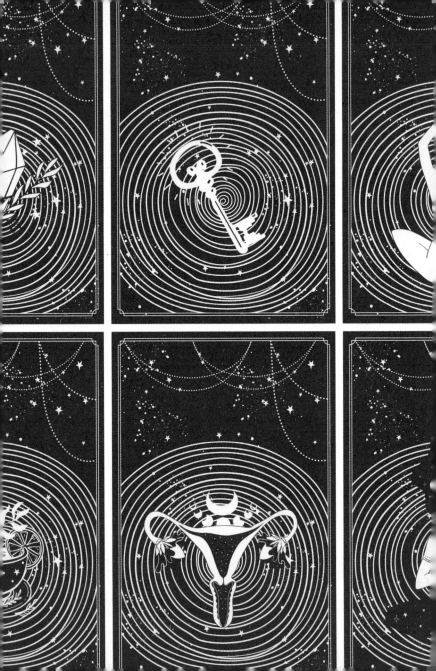

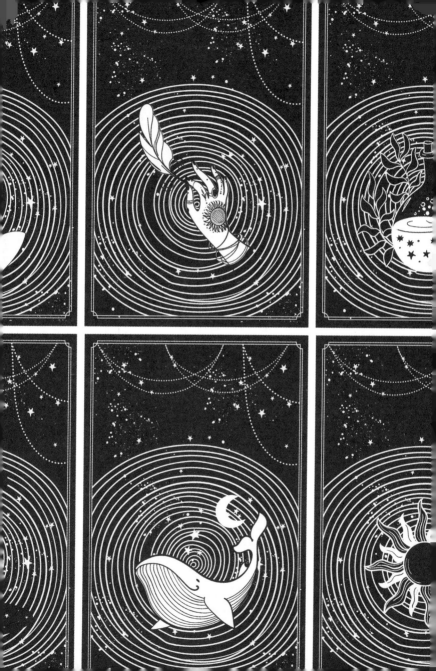

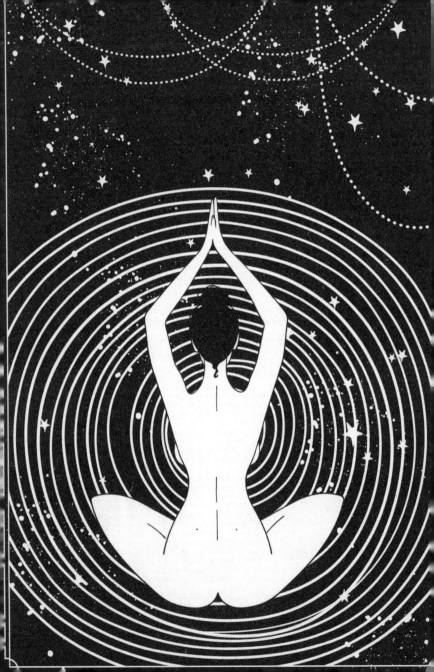

WOMB WITCH

HERBAL MAGICK FOR REPRODUCTIVE HEALTH

ANGELICA MERRITT

Microcosm Publishing
Portland, Ore | Cleveland, Ohio

WOMB WITCH: HERBAL MAGICK FOR REPRODUCTIVE HEALTH

© Angelica Merritt, 2025
© This edition Microcosm Publishing 2025
First edition - 3,000 copies - March 18, 2025
ISBN 9781648414572
This is Microcosm # 961
Cover by Lindsey Cleworth
Edited by Kandi Zeller
Design by Joe Biel

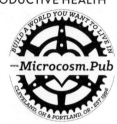

To join the ranks of high-class stores that feature Microcosm titles, talk to your rep: In the U.S. COMO (Atlantic), ABRAHAM (Midwest), BOB BARNETT (Texas, Oklahoma, Arkansas, Louisiana), IMPRINT (Pacific), TURNAROUND (UK), UTP/MANDA (Canada), NEWSOUTH (Australia/New Zealand), Observatoire (Africa, Europe), IPR (Middle East), Yvonne Chau (Southeast Asia), HarperCollins (India), Everest/B.K. Agency (China), Tim Burland (Japan/Korea), and FAIRE in the gift trade.

For a catalog, write or visit:
Microcosm Publishing
2752 N Williams Ave.
Portland, OR 97227

All the news that's fit to print at www.Microcosm.Pub/Newsletter

Get more copies of this book at www.Microcosm.Pub/WombWitch

For more witchy books, visit www.Microcosm.Pub/Witchy

Did you know that you can buy our books directly from us at sliding scale rates? Support a small, independent publisher and pay less than Amazon's price at **www.Microcosm.Pub.**

Global labor conditions are bad, and our roots in industrial Cleveland in the '70s and '80s made us appreciate the need to treat workers right. Therefore, our books are MADE IN THE USA.

MICROCOSM · PUBLISHING

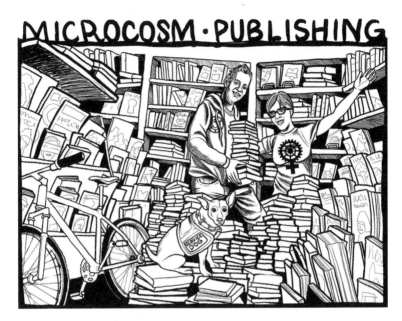

MICROCOSM PUBLISHING is Portland's most diversified publishing house and distributor, with a focus on the colorful, authentic, and empowering. Our books and zines have put your power in your hands since 1996, equipping readers to make positive changes in their lives and in the world around them. Microcosm emphasizes skill-building, showing hidden histories, and fostering creativity through challenging conventional publishing wisdom with books and bookettes about DIY skills, food, bicycling, gender, self-care, and social justice. What was once a distro and record label started by Joe Biel in a drafty bedroom was determined to be *Publishers Weekly*'s fastest-growing publisher of 2022 and #3 in 2023 and 2024, and is now among the oldest independent publishing houses in Portland, OR, and Cleveland, OH. We are a politically moderate, centrist publisher in a world that has inched to the right for the past 80 years.

Contents

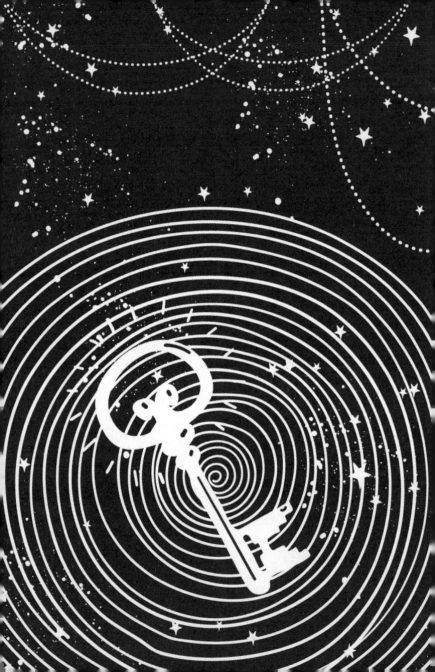

To body literacy for all. To know oneself is to free oneself.

Introduction

*A*re the inner workings of your body a mystery to you? Have you felt fear as politicians make nonsensical and dangerous laws about your uterus? You're not alone. This book exists to guide you as you find your power by embracing the womb witch within. Whether you have a uterus or love someone who does, the pages that follow offer a path toward autonomy through learning ancient knowledge and wisdom about the wombspace. While this knowledge has been smothered into an ember that's barely glowing within our western society, a spark remains, tended by the dedicated few.

The majority of us have not had the fortune to learn directly from the wisdom-keepers and elders who have kept this sage knowledge alive. This book acts as seeds from their pockets—seeds scattered into every sentence and meant to be tended to, reaped, and shared. On every page, these sprouts of knowledge are there to equip you with knowledge on your journey toward self-sovereignty.

In short, *Womb Witch* is a guidebook for those who long to be in touch with their wombspace in both spiritual and functional ways. I emphasize both, for these combined insights guide us into the intuitive knowing witchcraft begs us to hone. The womb is a sacred portal, a direct pathway into the life cycles of all that is. From it, the life-death-rebirth cycle is enacted. Through the process of getting to know the wombspace, we discover a deeper understanding of what is held inside of our bodies: magick and wonder. In this magick and wonder, we find the essence of witchcraft. But what exactly is a womb witch?

What Makes a Womb Witch?

Witchcraft has seen a strong renaissance in the past decade, with many reclaiming the word *witch* as an avowed path of self-empowerment. However, old definitions still linger—such as the one provided by Oxford Learners Dictionary, which describes a witch as a person "believed to have magic powers, especially to do evil things." This connotation does not resonate with the majority of witches and echoes the core of colonialism, which has historically demonized the practice of connecting with the cycles of nature, magick, and the deep reservoirs of intuition that lie within us all. It is this sacred connection that informs my understanding and practice of witchcraft, and it is in this spirit that this book is written.

There are many different paths and lineages of witchcraft, each with its own focus and direction. There are green witches, hedge witches, eclectic witches, kitchen witches, and on and on. How one witch presents and practices may vary largely from another. Likewise, my approach may differ from that of other witches. I believe womb witchcraft is not beholden to its own niche. The practices and information offered in this book are paramount for all witches to familiarize themselves with. If you do not house a womb, you came from one. Because of this, it is our responsibility to know the very basics of tending to ourselves and others in our community, for all of human life originates from this place. The health of wombs is intrinsically tied to the health of society.

Body literacy is the process of learning one's own natural rhythms, sensations, and reactions to foster awareness and understanding of one's personal health. This knowledge opens the door to radical reliance on caring for ourselves and others. It also shields us from the external forces that dictate our laws and education. The power of body literacy aligns seamlessly with the practice of witchcraft as both emphasize the importance of intuition, self-knowledge, and personal sovereignty.

Allow me to define womb witchcraft as I envision it throughout this book. While I do not claim this to be a definitive definition, it is what guided the insights and practices that follow. Remember, as with this entire book, take what resonates with you and leave the rest. I invite you to add your own nuances to this definition. Make it your own.

Womb witches…

- are deeply in touch with the natural rhythms and cycles of the body and nature
- place importance on connecting to their intuitive knowing
- use herbs, foods, practices, and rituals supportive of the wombspace
- see the connections: "as above and so below"[1]
- condemn restriction of knowledge and uplift the rite of sharing wisdom with the next generation
- exist as beings who see the sacred within themselves and each other

In short, womb witchery is for everyone who desires to connect to the power of knowledge and wisdom about and from the wombspace.

Who Is This Book For?

This book is for every womb and for everyone who longs to learn about the wombspace. There is no one who is not welcome here. I truly stand by the idea that it hurts no one to include everyone. Each page was crafted as an offering to any and every person who seeks its words for the betterment of themselves or those they love. In this vein, this information was crafted to

---

1 "As above and so below" is a phrase from *The Emerald Tablet*, a hermetic text, and refers to the microcosm and macrocosm. In essence, this phrase expresses the idea that what happens "above" on a larger scale is happening "below" on a smaller scale. It communicates the connection the spiritual world has to the material plane.

be shared: with your partner, your mom/parent, your sister/sibling, your neighbor, your best friend, and anyone else who you may encounter who may be helped by this knowledge. I invite you here even if you do not identify with the word witch, for that is by no means a requirement to read and implement this book.

Occasionally, you will see me using terminology like *women, woman, female, mother*. I would like to note that not all people who have wombs are women, and not all women have wombs. There are non-binary folks with wombs, trans men who have wombs, AFAB[2] people and women who do not have a womb from birth or who have had their wombs removed, just to name a few womb experiences. In this book, it is my deepest wish to welcome, celebrate, and represent the vast diversity of ways people with wombs can present. With all this in mind, I want to note that, within these pages, when I reference the reproductive system, I'm referring to the female reproductive system unless noted otherwise.

Why I'm Writing This Book

After I decided to stop taking birth control pills[3] in 2012, I dedicated myself to fertility awareness, which gave me the opportunity to learn about the intricacies of my body. What made me tick? What foods felt most nourishing throughout my cycle? When was I actually ovulating? Why did I experience overwhelming sensitivity before I started bleeding? These were questions I slowly found the answers to through self-study, my first herbal apprenticeship, and pouring over books on the subject of womb health.

2 AFAB is an acronym that stands for "assigned female at birth."

3 I started taking birth control pills at age 15 at the suggestion of my OB-GYN to lengthen my 16- to 18-day cycles. I realized I couldn't remember a time where I had not been on the pill and suspected these pills were causing disturbances I wasn't able to clearly detect while taking them. Within a year of stopping the pill, my body felt less inflamed and my emotions more manageable, and I had a clearer picture of my own intuitive guidance.

This great remembering of my relationship to my womb and womanhood allowed me to find my roots in herbalism, animism, and paganism, as well as through following and aligning myself with the Wheel of the Year. It saved me and baptized me in the waters of my innate wildness, from which I felt truly starved. With these new eyes, I saw that the sacred was everywhere as well as within me.

I steadily drifted into my path as a green witch. With my father a flower-loving landscaper and my grandfather a hobby farmer, I grew up in the dirt, planting seeds and dazzling over blooms and vegetables of all kinds. However, it wasn't until I had a handful of years away from my small-town, Christian upbringing that I understood that my authentic, personal beliefs and the way in which I experience the world was akin to being a witch. My deep, spiritual connection to the plant path was ignited during travels abroad when I was offered teas and oils as cures to my maladies. Returning home, I was changed and dedicated myself to learning about the plants in my bioregion and the rituals and wisdom of the Wheel of the Year.[4] But still, I had trepidation in claiming the identity of witch for fear of the judgment that would follow. The deep, healing connections I made with other women in a plant spirit apprenticeship I attended built up my confidence to fully accept this part of myself. My longing to seek solace within the natural world fused with my affinity for the mystical, and I've pursued this path unfailingly since.

Similarly to my journey with witchcraft, I discovered the power within my womb slowly, and then all at once. After experiencing an ectopic pregnancy while living abroad, I realized there was a vast gap in the knowledge I had when it came to my body. Despite practicing the fertility awareness method as a means of birth control for seven years, I did not know what

---

4 The Wheel of the Year marks the year's major solar events and includes the seasons, equinoxes, solstices, and midpoints between.

an ectopic pregnancy was or comprehend the severity of my condition for days. This situation put me in grave danger, and that experience propelled my path forward. I was hungry for knowledge, attending trainings on the wombspace and birth work and furthering my studies and practice in herbalism—all of which ultimately led to the scribing of these pages.

Along the way, I have pursued and embarked on thousands of hours of formal and informal studying, education, client work, and teaching within the realms of herbalism, energy work, full-spectrum pregnancy loss doula support, postpartum tending, breathwork, and kitchen witchery. Additionally, I graduated with a Bachelor of Science in Journalism from Ohio University, which assisted me greatly through the process of crafting and researching for this book.

What You'll Find in This Book

This book includes three parts. Part One introduces the basic concepts of the wombspace through overviews of wombspace anatomy, menstrual cycle awareness, and the womb life cycle (from puberty to menarche to menopause), as well as insights into the varying experiences a woman may have. As per the whole book, Part One incorporates elements of the magickal and the mundane. Rituals, archetypes, and accessible technical definitions are infused into each chapter.

Part Two provides a crash course on womb herbalism. It covers what herbalism is, herbal energetics, and important safety and best practices for working with herbs as a womb witch. Before administering herbs, it is imperative to have a practical understanding of this section.

In Part Three, we dive more deeply into specific herbs and holistic practices for tending to the wombspace. This will be where to find information on recipes, therapies, and preparations for the menstrual cycle, the womb life cycle, and many other different womb experiences.

There is no part of the book that is not related to the next and because of this, I highly recommend reading it in totality. For example, even if you have long passed the stage of puberty but know someone who may be experiencing puberty or will eventually experience this, I encourage you to continue by reading the information on puberty. This remains true for every section of the book. The information presented can be applied in various situations and can help all of us as we work together as a community and as womb witches.

Now, before we dive in more deeply, we turn to fundamental information and terms about witchcraft and womb health.

Foundational Terms and Concepts about Witchcraft and Womb Health

Throughout this book, I'll be mentioning some terms and concepts that may need a bit of introduction if you are new to witchcraft or womb health. Below are some brief definitions and ideas that undergird the foundations of this book and my womb witch practice.

Holistic Womb Health

Folk wisdom, which is the wisdom shared within the community, is what this book is heavily saturated in. In essence, this wisdom shows us how to live closer in alignment with our natural rhythms.

Holism is spiritual, emotional, physical, and mental—every part as important as the next. This book looks to enlighten you on each of these components with the hope that you ingrain what feels aligned into your life. The more we know HOW to work with our menstrual cycles and the overall cycle of life, the more empowered we are to show up in this world and in the human experience. This knowledge is the gift we can offer to those close to us, as well as to future generations.

The Wisdom-Keepers: A Brief History of Womb-Workers

This book would not be possible without the work of mothers, midwives/doulas/birth workers, feminists/activists, healthcare workers, and wisdom-keepers who have gingerly dedicated themselves to disseminating the old ways—the truth and power behind our wombs. Because of these people, we have this information available to learn and implement.

To properly attribute the sources from which I have learned a great deal of this information, we must review the history of midwifery and herbalism, in which much of this information is saturated in wisdom. Do note: This history is rich and extensive. My brief description of this history does not properly depict the dense and imperative knowledge these birth workers and herbalists honed in on and taught. If the information in this book offers you depth, I highly encourage the suggested reading material provided at the end of this book. This work would not be possible without those who dedicated their lives to preserving this knowledge and thus inspiring the grand majority of the studies and papers whose excerpts are featured.

Midwifery

Historically, those tending to birth and pregnancy were midwifery practitioners, women in the community who were experienced as dedicated healers and sources of wisdom for women and in pregnancy. It was common through the eighteenth and nineteenth centuries in the U.S. for birth to take place in one's home, surrounded by close family members, other women/womb-bearers, and birth workers.

Midwifery was practiced and taught by women who were enslaved, were Indigenous, and who had immigrated from Europe and Asia. Enslaved women who acted as birth workers were referred to as granny midwives.[5] They not only attended to the births of other enslaved women but also to slave-owner wives and other members of the local community, who they would be permitted to travel to.[6] These women were instrumental in imparting wisdom on not only birth but also birth control, abortion, and general womb health. With the medicalization of birth in the twentieth century by the self-imposed pedigree of white physicians, the U.S. society saw a bulk elimination of midwifery.[7] Midwifery was denounced and depicted as dangerous and unhygienic and considered to be practicing witchcraft/voodoo, which absolutely held a negative connotation at the time. Black midwives were purposefully excluded and demeaned from the movement to hospital births.[8] We must recognize the inherent racism and generational trauma incurred within this movement and practice, which was heightened with the Sheppard-Towner Maternity and Infancy Protection Act. This act was a seven-year government program passed in 1921, created to offer opportunities for education, medical care, and birth-worker training with certification, which was increasingly pushed as the only "legitimate" type of midwife.

At the time of this book being written, it is not currently legal in all fifty states in the U.S. for midwifery to be practiced. However, we are seeing an uptick in those choosing to use midwives and doulas in their birth team. According to the

5 National Museum of African American History and Culture, "The Historical Significance of Doulas and Midwives," February 1, 2022, nmaahc.si.edu/explore/stories/historical-significance-doulas-and-midwives.

6 "Historical Background," exhibits.mclibrary.duke.edu/duke-midwifery/historical-background/.

7 NIH, "Where Have All the Midwives Gone?," 2004, ncbi.nlm.nih.gov/pmc/articles/PMC2582410/.

8 Anika Nayak, "The History That Explains Today's Shortage of Black Midwives," *TIME*, February 29, 2024, time.com/6727306/black-midwife-shortage-history/.

U.S.Government Accountability Office, 12 percent of births in 2021 were attended to by midwives.[9]

Herbalism

Herbalism has existed for as long as humans and plants have existed in the same space. Even Neanderthals used plants in medicinal ways, showing we have always embraced herbs as remedies to that which ails us.[10]

Those in the realms of western, folk herbalism—as it is practiced in the U.S.—can largely give thanks for this knowledge to the Black, Indigenous, and immigrant people that kept this plant wisdom alive. *Womb Witch* incorporates a medley of plants, some of which were brought over by European settlers and enslaved people, some of which are native to the U.S., and some of which are herbs which are historically used in Ayurveda and Traditional Chinese Medicine (TCM). The herbs that are native to the lands of the U.S. were traditionally used by Indigenous people for centuries. Much of what we know about these plants was taught by these communities. Plants were seen not only as medicine to the physical body but also as spiritual guides and messengers, offering a soul-level connection that spanned beyond their scientific, medicinal aspects. Enslaved Black people brought herbal seeds with them across the middle passage, wearing these seeds as necklaces, which they then planted. These people not only served as midwives for their communities but also tended to the sick and made medicines from the plants which they brought and lived among. The enslaved and Indigenous communities were also known to share medicinal and spiritual

9 U.S. GAO, "Midwives: Information on Births, Workforce, and Midwifery Education," n.d., gao.gov/products/gao-23-105861#:~:text=Data%20show%20that%20in%202021,have%20increased%20in%20recent%20years.

10 Karen Hardy, Stephen Buckley, Matthew J. Collins, Almudena Estalrrich, Don Brothwell, Les Copeland, Antonio García-Tabernero, et al., "Neanderthal Medics? Evidence for Food, Cooking, and Medicinal Plants Entrapped in Dental Calculus," *Naturwissenschaften* 99, no. 8 (2012): 617–26, doi.org/10.1007/s00114-012-0942-0.

plant wisdom with each other.[11] European immigrants also brought with them plants from their bioregions. This history can be felt with the proliferation of Plantain (*Plantago spp.*), which was also referred to as "White Man's Footprint" by Native Americans. While herbalism is a field where information and the usage of plant medicine is shared and experienced, it is important to note that the knowledge of native and enslaved people was largely co-opted and claimed by white folks as their own.

In the nineteenth and early twentieth century, the Eclectics, a group of mostly male practitioners who practiced herbal medicine, fused European and Native American herbal medicine to offer an alternative to the usage of bloodletting and mercury, which both were popularized during this time by physicians. While the Eclectics were systematically shut down in the early 1900s, eventually a popularization of herbal medicine and home remedies saw a revival in the 60s and 70s.

Today, herbal medicine is slowly making its way into the mainstream as a more gentle, mostly side effect–free route to healing oneself. Herbal schools and businesses are popping up left and right and MDs are opening up to the idea of their patients using these medicines as legitimate ways to find holistic balance and through usage prophylactically. Herbalism is not only practiced by green witches but also by those who feel called to connect with the plant world in a meaningful way which intrinsically is tied to our ancestry.

After all, without plant medicine, we would not be here today.

---

11 Booker T. Washington, National Park Service, U.S. Department of the Interior, and Booker T. Washington National Monument, "Introduction," n.d., nps.gov/bowa/learn/historyculture/upload/the-final-plant-uses-site-bulletin.pdf.

Witchcraft

Every time this book is read or its information shared and practiced, it casts a spell that deeply participates in the wave of change. In its wake, my wish is that this book offers you a general understanding on how our bodies work, and how to tend to them naturally and magickally. The witchcraft elements in this book are infused into every chapter. The core components we will dive into include herbalism, rituals, archetypes, journaling, and holistic therapies—which all incorporate the elements which are infused in us all that exists on this planet: earth, wind, fire, water, and spirit. Let us touch on how each of these components will strengthen your practice of womb witchcraft.

Herbalism in Witchcraft

Herbalism is typically associated with the green witch path and the element of earth. But it is a practice that is open to every-witch and everyone that does not call themselves a witch. Through herbalism, we study the medicinal and magickal properties of wild flora. With these healing botanicals, we can create medicines, potions, sacred smokes, and rituals, which offer us a deeper connection with all of the elements. Herbalism is different from allopathic medicine and will not cause symptoms and root causes to disappear overnight. Plants do not act in the same way as pills, and it is important to keep this notion in mind when working with them. Mostly, they are slow-acting and require consistent use, depending on their nature and yours combined.

The herbs discussed in this book are mostly plants that are native or have found themselves in the United States. However, many of them grow on multiple continents, either due to their nature, through immigration, or through colonization. Above all, I believe that the plants that grow in your bioregion are the ones you should be working with. I have found these are the plants that will speak to our conditions and souls most deeply, offering medicine that is not only fresh but potent in the way it tends to us on a grounded level. I deeply respect, revere, and give credit to all I have learned from the plants themselves, as well as the wisdom I've learned through teachers of Native American, European, Ayurvedic, Traditional Chinese Medicine, and Black descent. Without these wisdom-keepers, this information would not be available to us, nor would the studies on these plants be inspired.

Rituals

Rituals are a means to connect the outer world and inner world, a pathway to spirit. The rituals in this book are not meant to be overly complicated, but they do require your full presence and respect if they are to work fruitfully. The majority of the crafted rituals will only require simple household and personal items. As I do not include specific crystals and stones within my practice, you will not see them suggested here. When readying yourself to enact a ritual, my suggestion is to read through the suggested sequence. Close your eyes and imagine what participating in this ritual will look like for you. From there, I encourage you to mold it into your own. This may look like incorporating varying objects, elements, or divination tools. Or, it may look like performing the ritual exactly as written. In all, I aimed to keep these rites simple, accessible, and easily accommodated for all bodies and all people who long to perform them.

Archetypes

Archetypes are recurrent symbols within society. Within the context of this book, we review the classic archetypes associated with the womb: Maiden, Mother, Crone. Working with archetypes is something humans have done for all of our history to bridge our connection to the patterns and roles we play within our human experience. They come to us in stories, mythology, the tarot, divination, Jungian psychology, and in every person we know. It's important to remember that nuance is present with every archetype. You may not identify with the specific name of the archetype, but implementing the overarching themes of these three specific archetypes is a way to infuse the process of knowing oneself through the mystical elements of the womb life cycle.

Journaling

It may strike you as curious to list journaling as a practice of witchcraft. But word witchery is something many—myself included—practice, for words are spells. There are several sections in this book with opportunities to answer prompts, ushering you into a deeper dive into its topic. This will allow you to excavate wells of information to steer you before, during, and/or after your ritual practice and bring you closer to occupying your body more fully.

Holistic Therapies

The holistic therapies reviewed throughout this book have a history of offering profound healing to those who implement them. They are not administered carelessly, but in a way that requires devoted attention. One must enter a space of awareness and grounding, opening up to the magick within the elements used. In moxibustion, we bring forth mugwort (earth), fire, and smoke (air) to encourage circulation, warmth, and stimulation. In breathwork, we welcome the element of air to bring ourselves into our bodies, further grounding ourselves into the earth. These therapies bring us closer to our magick and innate knowing. Where appropriate, I will take note of what communities are responsible for bringing us these practices.

Before Herbs, Addressing Our Lifestyle

Before we can move into using herbs for nourishment and support for any body and any situation, we must first address our lifestyle. Failing to do so will result in, well, poor results. Herbs are not prescription pills or band-aids to apply to exasperated situations. They can enhance environments that are ready for deep healing. For this to occur, diet, movement, sleep, and stress—which are oftentimes a large part of the root cause—must be considered.

This is why these elements are included when reviewing the phases of the menstrual cycle. It is instrumental to consider these factors, as they will greatly impact stress levels, hormone production, mental health, and ultimately, overall health. This is a part of the holistic framework. Even if you are not currently or will never again experience a menstrual cycle, this information can be applied and used for most bodies as a good place to start for movement and a nourishing diet. Of course, adjustments must be made for those who have specific health conditions and are pregnant and postpartum or breastfeeding.

A note on dieting before I discuss food choices: I am not at all an advocate for fad dieting. I am a proponent of finding foods that feel good, nourishing, and satisfying to one's body. There are no "bad" foods or "good" foods as what may be suitable for one person may cause food intolerances, allergies, or harsh reactions for another. There is no one diet to rule them all. Find a baseline that works for you and build from there. Allow yourself pleasure within the foods you eat.

If I had to dish out one sentence that would summarize what all bodies would function the best on, it would be this: Focus on fresh foods. If you're focusing on fresh foods, it will be that much easier to get your daily needs of protein, fiber, healthy fats, and other recommended nutrients. However, for the basics of what that entails, here are my recommendations for what to look for when considering what types of foods to consume daily:

- Organic, pasture-raised, local meats and eggs
- Wild-caught seafood
- If you can incorporate wild foods into your diet, do so
- Organic dark, leafy greens, and colorful root veggies and squashes
- Organic berries and citrus
- Soaked and sprouted grains, nuts, and beans
- Small amounts of fermented foods
- Healthy fats (avocado, olive, coconut oils, ghee, grass-fed butter)

This list may seem like a long shot to incorporate into your life. And possibly even laughable due to the cost of buying food of this caliber, as well as the time it takes to prepare meals. These are simply suggestions with the overarching theme to do the best you can. I stress the importance of whole food sources as these are incredibly impactful for the transition phases in our lives. The shifts in life—menarche, pregnancy/postpartum, perimenopause/menopause—go much more smoothly when meals include enough protein, fat, and fiber-rich vegetables. Oftentimes, as we are growing, changing, and shifting, our bodies will be craving deep nutrition, which can be mistaken for "something dense," resulting in carb-heavy snacks and meals. There is nothing wrong with partaking in eating these things with balance. But, it is essential to consider what the body is saying by craving these things. A craving for salt may be linked to dehydration or stress. A craving for chocolate during or before bleeding may indicate a need for magnesium. A sugar craving may be a telltale sign that one's energy is lagging, physically or mentally, and can indicate a need for bitter foods, which balance one's desire for overly sweet foods.

Daily movement is another factor addressed in this book as movement equals circulation. Circulation means our body's pathways of elimination (sweating, urination, defecation) remain open and flowing. Our bodies were made to move with regularity, and a baseline of active movement ensures that our bodies remain healthy and functioning with ease. Per the American Heart Association, 150 minutes of moderate to intense exercise per week or 75 minutes of intense exercise per week, is the general recommendation. Balance is key here, as is finding movement that feels good and supportive to your body.

Another lifestyle factor we must consider is stress. Many of us experience an abundance of stress. We are constantly bombarded with an influx of messages, sounds, stimuli, and not-pleasant news. We are parents, sisters/siblings, caretakers, holders of many jobs, running households, and tending to our communities.

We can't all quit our jobs and relinquish the responsibilities that come along with raising a family or showing up in society. But, I do believe there are little things we can do to make our nervous systems run at a less frantic space through prioritizing extracurricular activities that build us up and nourishing our mental and physical bodies with practices that rejuvenate and restore.

Final Notes for the Journey

Before embarking on the journey of reading this book, please fully digest this statement: Not all of this information will be for you, nor should all of it be applied to you.

This book is an invitation to learn the basic intricacies of taking care of the female body.

I am a clinical herbalist and doula, not a physician or a licensed medical professional. Do not consider this book a prescription or a command. Womb Witch is an accumulation of information I have gathered over years of study, through implementation in my own and clients' lives, from books, articles, and scientific papers, as well as things I have learned through teachers I trust far and wide. Before implementing a new practice, herb, or lifestyle shift, it is imperative that you do extra research to ensure you do not have a contraindicated medical condition or take a prescription pill that would be affected. Please consult a health practitioner if you are unsure if any of these things are not right for you to try.

As you go through these pages, the sheer amount of information being presented can be overwhelming. However, remember this: Your life routines do not need to change all at once, or at all if something doesn't feel aligned. However, if a practice written here feels aligned or invigorating or makes you curious, I do encourage you to consider trying it.

A golden rule when learning new material: Be gentle with yourself, be patient, and be consistent. Consider saying these phrases aloud and writing them down: Be gentle. Be patient. Be consistent with whatever you decide to try.

Don't expect a miracle overnight. Remind yourself that you are learning something we should have been taught as we grew into our adult bodies. This can be frustrating. It's also really exciting. Even though many of us did not have this information when we were younger, we can implement these practices now. We can live a more vibrant, present, and aware life while preventatively taking care of our bodies in the present. This is the gift of body literacy.

Part One: Anatomy of the Wombspace

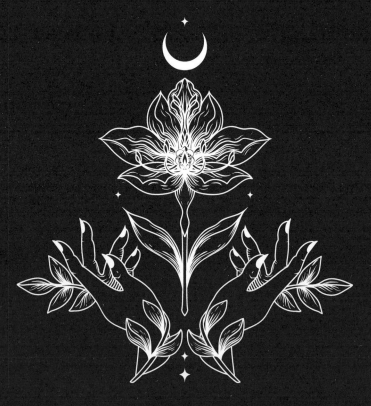

Introduction

*H*ave you ever touched your cervix? Do you know what your labia is? How would you describe where your vagina is and what it encompasses? Are you aware of the phases of your menstrual cycle? Do you know about the life cycle of the womb, from puberty to menopause? Have you had the opportunity to learn about womb experiences commonly left out of the conversation, like PCOS, endometriosis, or pregnancy loss? This is information not expressed or taught to many outside of the medical community. And so this basic knowledge must be reviewed, reframed, and made available as points of reference, which we will do in the chapters that follow in this section

In Chapter One, we'll cover the basic anatomical parts of the wombspace, as well as the hormones involved there. Chapter Two is a review of the menstrual cycle phases and their adjacent supportive holistic tools. In Chapter Three, we'll look at the life cycle of the womb through the lens of the archetypes Maiden, Mother, and Crone. Finally, Chapter Four delves into other womb experiences that are often silenced or sidelined. Reminder: We will not be discussing herbal medicine in this part of the book.

Together, let's embark on a journey of autonomy through learning about the anatomy and accompanying experiences of the wombspace.

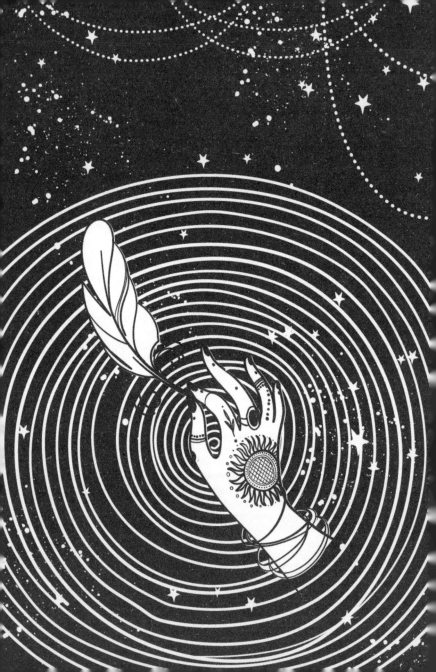

Chapter One: The Parts of the Wombspace

hile practitioners and those who yearn for deep dives into what they are learning would love a long descriptor for each of the anatomical and physiological parts of the wombspace, I've opted for a lighter approach. For the sake of keeping this information accessible, I've chosen simple and non-intimidating reviews of anatomy, as well as a section on hormones that play a large role in the wombspace.

Each part and function of the reproductive system could command multiple books. Here, we are looking for reference points. Easy descriptors. A tidy paragraph offering sufficient understanding. If you leave these pages wanting more, I invite you to seek the resources at the end of the book, which will aid you in further educating yourself if you feel inspired.

As you read this overview of the womb-based reproductive system, contemplate where each is in your body. If you have never before done so, fetch a mirror and look at your external anatomy as you review its name and function. Consider putting your hand over each internal area as you read about it to play out the mind-body connection. Feel the power from within. Learning about ourselves in this way is an important step in body literacy, autonomy, and unveiling the magick that awaits its unleashing.

Anatomical Parts of the Wombspace

Breasts

While your breasts do not directly enact the menstruation process, they are deeply connected to other reproductive organs. Breasts are the glandular organs located on the chest which contain connective tissue, fat, and breast tissue. Breast tissue contains mammary glands which produce milk. Breasts are sensitive to hormone changes and participate in the cyclical, monthly phases our bodies undergo. They not only provide nourishment to babies but also can function for arousal.

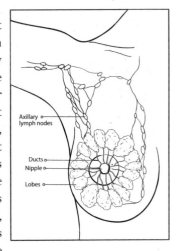

Uterus

The uterus is one place we have all lived as a collective, as this is where the gestation of babies occurs. It is pear-shaped and located between the bladder and rectum. The uterus is extremely important in hormone regulation, as it is connected to the ovaries.

Ovaries

As detailed above, the ovaries are connected to each side of the uterus. They are endocrine-secreting glands which are each the size and shape of an almond. Ovaries are responsible for secreting hormones and preparing eggs for ovulation/fertilization. They also play a very important role in maintaining health and vitality into menopause. Some of the hormones produced and secreted by the ovaries are progesterone and estrogen, as well

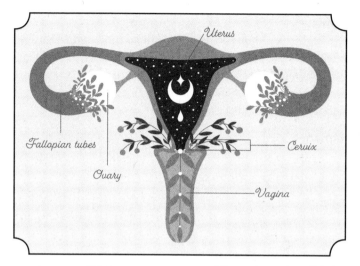

Uterus

Fallopian tubes

Ovary

Cervix

Vagina

as androgens. All the eggs someone will ever have in a lifetime are present in the ovaries from birth.

Fallopian Tubes

The fallopian tubes are located in the mesosalpinx, which is the outer tissue layer that wraps around the tubes and is a component of the uterus.[12] On average, these organs are 10 to 12 cm in length and are lined with a mucous membrane that aids in the transportation of eggs and sperm to the uterine cavity. They also are what connects the ovaries to the uterus.

Cervix

At the very bottom of the uterus is the cervix. It is what connects the uterus to the vagina through a small opening. The varying cervical fluid experienced throughout a menstrual cycle is produced here in a small group of cells in the cervix called the endocervical gland cells.

12 Joan Han and Nazia M. Sadiq, "Anatomy, Abdomen and Pelvis: Fallopian Tube," StatPearls - NCBI Bookshelf, July 24, 2023, ncbi.nlm.nih.gov/books/NBK547660/#:~:text=Fallopian%20tubes%2C%20otherwise%20called%20oviducts,terminate%20near%20the%20ipsilateral%20ovary.

Vagina

The vagina is a mucous membrane-lined tube that connects to the cervix and vulva. It is considered "the gateway to life," as it is the channel by which many babies are born. It is also the place where sperm start their travel for possible fertilization. Menstrual blood and cervical fluid are excreted from here.

Hymen

The hymen is a tissue located at the opening of the vagina that is left over from fetal development. It serves no purpose in the menstruation process or the health of your wombspace. Hymens present in many different sizes and shapes. And contrary to popular belief, the hymen does not provide proof of whether someone has had sex or not.[13]

Vulva

The vulva encompasses the genitalia located outside of a body with a womb, which includes the opening of the vagina, the urethral opening, the clitoris, the labia majora/minora, Bartholin's glands, and mons pubis.

The clitoris is located at the top of the vulva. It fills with blood when aroused, which is the same way a penis becomes erect. This spot contains more sexual nerve endings than any other part of the body. In total, the clitoris is 5 inches long. If you have one, it's also what you may be able to thank for a grand majority of your orgasms, as a staggering percentage of women can only climax with clitoral stimulation.

The urethral opening is located between the clitoris and the opening of the vagina. This is where urination is expelled.

Near the vaginal opening are the Bartholin's glands, which are responsible for producing lubrication during sexual arousal. The labia majora and minora are the lips that protect the vaginal opening. The labia majora is the outer skin fold where pubic

13 "Hymen," Cleveland Clinic, n.d., my.clevelandclinic.org/health/body/22718-hymen.

hair grows, while the labia minora are inside of the majora and connected to the clitoris. Lastly, the mons pubis is the rounded area in front of the pubic bone and directly above your vulva.

Hormones and Other Important Parts of the Wombspace

Cholesterol

If you're unfamiliar with sex steroid hormone production, cholesterol—since it is not a hormone itself—may be a surprising item to find on a list of sexual reproductive hormones. While cholesterol plays an active role in many areas throughout the body, it is the predecessor of all sex hormones. Cholesterol turns into pregnenolone.

Pregnenolone

Pregnenolone is the precursor for all steroid hormones, including progesterone, androgens, estrogen, and testosterone. Maintaining a balanced level of pregnenolone is essential for overall hormonal health.

Progesterone

Progesterone is a sexual reproductive hormone produced and secreted by the ovaries, as well as the adrenal cortex.[14] It aids in regulating the menstrual cycle and readies the uterus for pregnancy by thickening the lining of the uterus in preparation for a fertilized egg.[15]

Androgens

While many people think of male reproductive hormones when they consider androgens, it's important to note that they are

14 Lane K. Christenson and Luigi Devoto, "Cholesterol transport and Steroidogenesis by the Corpus Luteum," *Reproductive Biology and Endocrinology: RB&E* 90, no. 1 (2003), ncbi.nlm.nih.gov/pmc/articles/PMC280730/.
15 Jessie K. Cable and Michael H. Grider, "Physiology, Progesterone," StatPearls - NCBI Bookshelf, May 1, 2023, ncbi.nlm.nih.gov/books/NBK558960/.

also produced and used for important things in the female body. The primary androgen is testosterone. Androgens aid in some of the effects of puberty and assist in the function of ovarian health, among many other things.

Estrogen

Estrogen is one set of sexual reproductive hormones that are mostly produced by the ovaries, although it can also be produced in fat cells as well as in the adrenal glands. Included in this group are estradiol, estrone, and estriol. Estrogen regulates the menstrual cycle and guides the development of sexual reproductive organs/puberty. It affects not only the sexual reproductive system but many organ systems, including the brain and musculoskeletal systems.

Follicle Stimulating Hormone

Follicle Stimulating Hormone, referred to as FSH, is produced in the pituitary gland. This hormone is a part of the development of reproductive systems and aids in controlling the menstrual cycle. Specifically, it triggers the production of eggs in the ovaries, readying them for ovulation.[16]

Luteinizing Hormone

Luteinizing Hormone (LH) is also produced in the pituitary gland and is a hormone that helps with the development of the reproductive system. LH regulates the menstrual cycle 17by stimulating steroid hormone production which enacts processes such as ovulation and menstruation.[18]

16 "Follicle-Stimulating Hormone (FSH) Levels Test," n.d., medlineplus.gov/lab-tests/follicle-stimulating-hormone-fsh-levels-test/#:~:text=FSH%20plays%20an%20important%20role,the%20eggs%20ready%20for%20ovulation.

17 PubMed, "Physiology, Luteinizing Hormone," January 1, 2024, pubmed.ncbi.nlm.nih.gov/30969514/#:~:text=In%20men%2C%20LH%20causes%20the,an%20egg%20in%20the%20uterus%20.

18 Daniel Nedresky and Gurdeep Singh, "Physiology, Luteinizing Hormone," StatPearls - NCBI Bookshelf, September 26, 2022, ncbi.nlm.nih.gov/books/NBK539692/#article-24535.s5.

Chapter Two: Menstrual Cycle Awareness

The Menstrual Cycle

*T*he menstrual cycle is a cyclical, life-death pattern the body experiences from the onset of menarche until menopause. An egg is released, and the uterus prepares to possibly receive a fertilized egg. If fertilization does not occur, the uterine lining is shed and a new cycle begins. This process is the microcosm to the macrocosm of the entire life cycle of a womb-being.

The typical menstrual cycle occurs every 19 to 32 days. This, of course, can shift depending on birth control methods, stress, and other health factors. There are three technical phases of the menstrual cycle, which include the follicular, ovulatory, and luteal phases. However, menstruation is largely considered its own phase, with the menstrual phase at the beginning of the follicular phase.

From a witchcraft perspective, these four phases are correlated to each season of the year. I've found applying the familiarity of the Wheel of the Year to the specific phase of the cycle eases the process of shifting into a more harmonic rhythm with one's body while moving away from our society's model of "Go, go, go" no matter the season. The moon phases have also historically been associated with menstruation, which I will touch on lightly in the pages to come.

It's important to remember that each of our bodies is unique. As such, each person's menstrual cycle will have differing experiences and needs. However, there are general needs the menstruating body has. For each phase of the cycle, there are varying foods, herbs, supplements, and movements that have been researched and historically used as a means to best support and nourish us.

This part of the book will give you an introductory level of information about each of the four phases of the cycle, along with foods, herbs, and movements and spiritual practices to invoke a closer connection to each phase.

I want to make an important note: there is no dogma present in these suggestions or pages. They are just that. Suggestions. Information. Research. Scientific studies. Cultural practices. Things that have worked for myself, my clients, and many others for many centuries. I implore you to use this guide not as a rulebook but as information on ways you may be able to better support your body.

I hope that looking more deeply and closely at the way we tend to ourselves will spark further insight not only in our physical realm but also in spiritual ways. Your connection with yourself is a sacred bond that should be protected and preserved. When you discover tools to understand and take care of yourself, it is a rewarding process that will allow you to feel safe, secure, and confident.

It may seem like foregoing a few glasses of wine while you're bleeding or eating a carrot salad post-ovulation won't offer such potency. But I've witnessed such small acts transform how we can exist and participate in our relationship with ourselves. I invite you to consider these small acts.

The Fertility Awareness Method and the Menstrual Cycle

Before we dive into talk about the menstrual cycle itself, I wanted to touch on one great tool in my own learning process: the Fertility Awareness Method (or FAM for short). Maybe you, the reader, are a person who has dreamt of being a mother or parent your whole life. Maybe you're unsure of what your stance is on bringing life into the earth. Or, maybe, you are fully aware you have no interest in procreating. Whatever way you splice it, being aware of the intimate ebbs and flows of your cycles is an important way to tune into your internal self.

Your fertility, whether you choose to use it or not, is an indicator of health. Learning about this method will allow you to assess the timing of each phase, preparing you in the ways you want to eat, move, and nourish yourself. And this process will also instill you with deeper wisdom and knowingness of the rhythms within.

The Fertility Awareness Method (FAM) is used for natural birth control/planning/body literacy and is one of the most recommended and precise forms of natural birth control. With that being said, it is interactive and will require full participation and awareness from those who choose this route.

As this method does require daily attention, it is certainly not for everyone. I, as always, encourage you to do what is best for you, your body, and your lifestyle. However, if you are looking for a new method of birth control, this is an extremely empowering and effective option.

There are three different methods of charting your fertility signs in FAM. They include charting cervical fluid, the position of your cervix, and your daily, waking basal body temperature (BBT)—all data that can be used to create a chart of a person's menstrual cycle. You can use these methods individually or together. However, ovulation CAN shift from cycle to cycle and year to year, so it is greatly recommended that you use all three methods to get a conclusive snapshot as to when you are/aren't fertile. With this in mind, it's necessary to mention that phone apps geared around tracking the menstrual cycle, which may try to predict your fertile window, will likely not be a trustworthy source of information.

As you can see, FAM is complex and deserves its own class: There are many such classes available, as well as books and zines, which is where I first encountered this practice. If you are interested in how you can begin utilizing the methods of FAM, I encourage you to pay attention and play along with the information shared on these pages. I will be going over what each phase of cervical fluid/cervical position signals and how to go about tracking them.

For each phase of the menstrual cycle that we go over, you will find corresponding information on cervical fluid and position patterns associated with that phase. If you are confused as to what cervical fluid you are looking at or experiencing, I recommend using some of the resources I've provided in the appendix. When tracking cervical fluid, it is recommended to practice abstinence for the first cycle as arousal and seminal fluid can mix with cervical fluid, complicating results and observations.

In addition to tracking your cervical fluid, I highly suggest charting Basal Body Temperature (BBT) as well. However, I will not be covering BBT on these pages. While it is theoretically possible to use cervical fluid tracking alongside Luteinizing Hormone strips as a means to predict fertility when used perfectly, it does not come without risks and should be treated as such. Allow me to stress this: Please do not use cervical fluid and position tracking as your only means of birth control if you are not including BBT, charting, and/or have extended your education and knowledge in this method.

With that being said, it is important to note that what I review in these pages is NOT sufficient enough to use as a sole method of birth control as nuance exists within each person and each cycle. I repeat: learn more about this birth control method before using it as your sole means of birth control. There is much I do not cover that is integral to this method being effective.

These practices take, well, practice. And, they are not to be used like the pill. True body literacy requires time to study, observe, and record…on repeat.

Charting Your Cervical Fluid/Positioning

To get started with tracking cervical fluid, you will be observing the cervical fluid present at the vulva or cervix.

As you begin, I suggest always checking fluid at the cervix. This will ensure you get an accurate picture of what you are observing as there will be more fluid present near the cervix as this is where the fluid comes from. Be sure to consistently check fluid from the same body position as this will allow you to get an accurate reading of the cervix position. The positioning of your cervix changes from one phase of the cycle to the next. Squatting, sitting on the toilet, or placing a leg on a tub to check are all great ways to start.

Things that may affect accurately assessing cervical fluid include lubricants, sexual activity (which will create arousal fluid that can sometimes be mistaken for ovulation fluid), spermicides, antihistamines, vaginal infections, hormonal birth control, fertility medications, alcohol, and expectorants. Do not underestimate these factors! Consider them as you are charting your cycles.

To assess your cervical fluid, wash your hands, insert two clean fingers into the vagina and gently push them back into the vaginal canal until you reach your cervix. Lightly, with a swooping, scissor-like motion, trap cervical fluid between your fingers and pull them out to observe. Rub the fluid between the thumb and pointer finger and note its consistency. We will review what the varying consistencies mean in the coming pages.

After you have practiced this for a full cycle, you can choose to observe your cervical fluid at the vulva or continue to observe it at the cervix. However, it is important to note that consistency is key. Choose where you would like to observe your fluid and stick with it.

In each menstrual cycle phase we discuss, I'll also mention the positioning of the cervix during each specific phase There are four descriptors used to chart the cervical positioning:

- Softness
- Height
- Opening
- Wetness

This is also referred to as SHOW. The softness of your cervix will be described as firm, medium, or soft. The height of your cervix will be described as low, middle, or high. The opening of your cervix will be described as closed, partly open, or high. The wetness of your cervix will be described as dry/nothing, sticky, creamy, or wet. The positioning will aid you as an additional sign in recognizing when you are fertile and whether or not ovulation is taking place.

A Note on Hormonal Birth Control

Hormonal birth control is an option many choose as a means to prevent pregnancy and may be prescribed to curb health symptoms that arise at the onset of menstruation such as acne, endometriosis cramps, short or long cycles, and PMS. When taking hormonal birth control, the body will respond by preventing ovulation, creating thicker cervical fluid which blocks sperm from entering the cervix and may also thin the lining of the uterus, which creates a hostile environment for a fertilized egg to grow. This form of birth control is 99 percent effective when used perfectly.[19] Long-term use of birth control has been found to increase the risk of breast and cervical

---

19 "Birth Control Pills," Cleveland Clinic, n.d., my.clevelandclinic.org/health/treatments/3977-birth-control-the-pill

cancer,[20] systemic inflammation,[21] and psychological disorders related to mood.[22]

While birth control is often prescribed by physicians for the symptoms described above and beyond, it is important to note that this does not mean the imbalance, or root cause, is being addressed. Rather, it may be being masked. I support folks with their choice in birth control methods or use as long as they are informed of these facts and what it means from a holistic lens.

The Moon Cycle and Our Wombs

The moon rotates around the Earth every 28 days. In this time, we experience a new moon, waxing crescent, first quarter, waxing gibbous, full moon, waning gibbous, third quarter, and a waning crescent. Slowly, the moon turns from dark to illuminated to dark again, enacting a similar dance as our cervixes and energetic bodies do throughout the menstrual cycle.

Our ancestors recognized and celebrated this similarity, knowing that, just as farmers plant seeds and tend to their gardens by the cycles of the moon, we can find wisdom in recognizing the natural cycles within ourselves and doing the same. The process of following the moon cycles in accordance with the womb is a spiritual practice that is not solely reserved for those who bleed. If you are a person with a womb who does not experience menstrual bleeding or has undergone menopause,

20 "Oral Contraceptives and Cancer Risk," National Cancer Institute, n.d., cancer.gov/about-cancer/causes-prevention/risk/hormones/oral-contraceptives-fact-sheet.

21 Summer Mengelkoch, Jeffrey Gassen, George M. Slavich, and Sarah E. Hill(2024). "Hormonal Contraceptive Use Is Associated with Differences in Women's Inflammatory and Psychological Reactivity to an Acute Social Stressor," Brain Behavior and Immunity 115, 747–757, doi.org/10.1016/j.bbi.2023.10.033.

22 Sarah Martell, Christina Marini, Cathy A. Kondas, and Allison B. Deutch, "Psychological Side Effects of Hormonal Contraception: A Disconnect between Patients and Providers," Contraception and Reproductive Medicine 8 (2023), doi.org/10.1186/s40834-022-00204-w.

I encourage you to work with the moon's cycles through the inner and outer work suggested in the passages where these cycles are discussed. We are cyclical beings with complex inner workings—whether or not ovulation, menstruation, or any other bodily process unfolds with regularity or at all.

As we discuss the phases of the menstrual cycle in the pages to come, I will include the moon phase associated with each one.

The Four Phases of the Menstrual Cycle

The four phases of the menstrual cycle command four unique time periods in the body, as we will learn.Here, we'll cover what specifically happens in the body during each phase, with special attention given to cervical fluid and position. Insights on food and movement guidance are offered as a means to empower you to embrace the rhythm of the wombspace in a way that works best for you. And since this is a guide for the whole person, each of the four phases also include spiritual insight sections, from corresponding moon phases to rituals to journal prompts. With all that in mind, let's journey together through the cycle of the womb!

Menstrual Phase (Days 1–7)

The first day of your menstrual cycle is the first day you are fully bleeding. Let's get that straight: It is not the last day you bleed, or the day you start spotting, but the first day you have a full flow of blood. That day is considered DAY ONE of your cycle. When you start bleeding, your previous cycle ends.

If the egg your body has prepared is not fertilized, your body sheds of thickened uterine lining, which is what creates the blood during your period. This is also the time where the hormones estrogen and progesterone drop.

The bleeding portion of the menstrual phase typically lasts between 2 to 7 days, but, as previously mentioned, may vary.

This is technically the beginning of the follicular phase but is also referred to as the menstrual phase.

In this phase, the body is working very hard and energy is at its lowest. Feeling introspective and withdrawn is a natural part of this phase. Your body is clearing out what is no longer needed so that it can make room for a new cycle. This encourages a process of slowing down to allow the body to recover. Take extra care to nourish the body with nourishing food and herbs, and place intention on keeping stress at a minimum.

With this in mind, it may come as no surprise that the menstrual/early follicular phase is the womb's winter season. Take a moment to consider the quiet calm that begets winter months: The bears are hibernating. The trees and plants are sending their energy into their roots. The birds have fled or are nesting, preserving their precious energy. In a similar way, the menstrual phase demands selfishness by way of prioritizing tending to yourself above all: as the rest taken here offers restoration for the duration of the cycle. Put another way, the menstrual phase invites us to tend to our roots, allowing for the expansion that takes place in the days and weeks after. This phase also prepares fertile ground for the seasons that follow.

Cervical Fluid / Position Menstrual

During the menstrual phase, you are bleeding, which means there is no cervical fluid present. Your cervix will be firm, low, and closed.[23]

Movement

To encourage rest, it is optimal to minimize, or the least, soften, your activities during the menstrual phase. Focus on gentle movement such as yin/restorative yoga, light walking, and

23 S. Parenteau-Carreau and C. Infante-Rivard, "Self-Palpation to Assess Cervical Changes in Relation to Mucus and Temperature," *International Journal of Fertility*, 33 (1988), 10-6, pubmed.ncbi.nlm.nih.gov/2902020/

stretching. This is typically not the time to do vigorous hikes, distance running, boot camp workouts, or day-long trips where you are excessively on your feet. Those more intense types of activities make you more prone to further exhausting your body, which can lead to chronic fatigue if done consistently from cycle to cycle.

However, different people in different bodies may find that more movement during the menstrual phase assists them in alleviating menstrual cramps, headaches, and fatigue. Only you will know how to proceed during this time. Be aware of how your body is truly feeling with a varying degree of movement.

NOTE: As we continue, you may find it beneficial to view the entirety of your cycle as one workout. There is a time for warming up (menstrual phase); the actual, heavy exercise portion (late follicular/ovulatory/early luteal phases); and a time for cooling down (late luteal phase/start of the next cycle).

Food

When bleeding, the body loses important nutrients which we aim to resupply through supportive food and herbs. This makes it important to properly nourish our bodies during the menstrual phase by focusing on eating foods that are rich in protein, fats,and omega-3s, as well as fresh vegetables/fruit and carbs that are high in fiber. It is also important to replenish stores of minerals and iron, which are lost through the blood.

When we are bleeding, the last thing many of us want to worry about is preparing food. This is where meal prepping can be instrumental. If there is any time in the cycle when relying on premade meals is optimal, it is during the menstrual phase. Consider keeping nutrient-dense and satisfying foods on hand in easy-to-eat and creative ways. Explore food blogs that resonate with your taste, time constraints, and accessibility needs. Additionally, having a list of restaurants that offer nutritious take-out options can be beneficial. If there is any time during your cycle you should feel entitled to rest, it is during this phase.

For this phase, supportive foods are rich in the following nutrients:

- B vitamins, which assist the body in using energy-rich nutrients and enzymes[24]
- Vitamin C, which promotes iron absorption and white blood cell production[25]
- Zinc, which remineralizes blood, supports a healthy immune system, and is a major part of the growth of cells[26]
- Omega-3 fatty acids, which lower overall inflammation and encourage a healthy mental space[27, 28]
- Magnesium, which is responsible for hundreds of processes within the body and is known to ease everything from period cramps to mental fatigue to allowing the body to rest more deeply[29]

Warming, slow-cooked foods will be especially nourishing to the body during this time.

As the body is undergoing a lot and clearing out quite a bit, it is best to avoid foods that will bring forth distress. (We go

24 The Nutrition Source, "B Vitamins," March 7, 2023, hsph.harvard.edu/nutritionsource/vitamins/vitamin-b/.

25 Sean R. Lynch and James D. Cook, "Interaction of Vitamin C and Iron," *Annals of the New York Academy of Sciences* 355, no. 1 (December 1, 1980): 32–44, doi.org/10.1111/j.1749-6632.1980.tb21325.x.

26 The Nutrition Source. "Zinc," March 7, 2023. hsph.harvard.edu/nutritionsource/zinc/#:~:text=It%20is%20a%20major%20player,childhood%2C%20adolescence%2C%20and%20pregnancy.

27 Seema Mehdi, Kishor Manohar, Atiqulla Shariff, Nabeel Kinattingal, Shahid Ud Din Wani, Sultan Alshehri, Mohammad T. Imam, Faiyaz Shakeel, and Kamsagara L. Krishna, "Omega-3 Fatty Acids Supplementation in the Treatment of Depression: An Observational Study," *Journal of Personalized Medicine* 13, no. 2 (January 27, 2023): 224, doi.org/10.3390/jpm13020224.

28 Artemis P. Simopoulos, "Omega-3 Fatty Acids in Inflammation and Autoimmune Diseases," *Journal of the American College of Nutrition* 21, no. 6 (December 1, 2002): 495–505, doi.org/10.1080/07315724.2002.10719248.

29 "Office of Dietary Supplements - Magnesium," n.d., ods.od.nih.gov/factsheets/Magnesium-HealthProfessional/.

into that further below.) Cravings tend to be at an all-time high when bleeding. If you're experiencing extreme symptoms when menstruating, it may be helpful to review the following list of supportive foods to see how you may be able to support your body by eliminating or adding certain foods.

Supportive Foods for the Menstrual / Early Follicular Phase

- Meat/Poultry/Seafood/Protein: Wild-Caught Salmon, Mussels, Grass-Fed Beef, Free-Range Chicken/Turkey/ Eggs, Wild-Caught Tuna, Organic Tofu (Firm & Sprouted), Halibut, Cod, Mackerel, Oysters, Lobster, Shrimp, Clams
- Vegetables: Sweet Potatoes, Acorn Squash, Butternut Squash, Tomatoes, Broccoli, Bell Pepper, Collard Greens, Kale, Chard, Beets, Carrots
- Fruits: Strawberries, Kiwi, Papaya, Avocado, Oranges, Lemon, Lime, Grapefruit, Cantaloupe, Black Cherries
- Legumes/Nuts/Grains (Soaked & Sprouted): Almonds, Pumpkin Seeds, Sesame Seeds, Lentils, Garbanzo Beans, Quinoa, Oats, Hemp Seeds
- Dairy/Non-Dairy: Yogurt (Grass-Fed Full Fat/Greek Yogurt or Organic Coconut Yogurt)
- Oils/Fats: Avocado Oil, Unrefined Coconut Oil, Cold Pressed Extra Virgin Olive Oil, Sesame Oil, Hemp Oil, Grass-Fed Ghee/Butter
- Other: Seaweed, Himalayan Sea Salt, Bone Broth, Organic Almond Butter, Dark Chocolate

Foods to Avoid during the Menstrual Phase

The foods listed here are typically heavy on the body and energetically intense, making them less than ideal for this phase of rest. While I suggest avoiding these types of food (or at least keeping them to a minimum) while you are bleeding, do not treat this list as a rulebook. Diet culture is toxic and not welcome in these pages. Every body is different, and the food suggestions are meant to act as supportive guides and informational insight into possible root causes of imbalances.

- *Processed, fried foods* are laden with Omega-6-rich seed oils and preservatives, which are thought to increase inflammation in the body and cause gut disturbance, especially when adequate amounts of Omega-3 fatty acids are missing from the diet.[30]
  - » Consider replacing them with foods cooked in an air fryer. Baked sweet potato fries. Premade, homemade foods such as sourdough pancakes or protein muffins.
- *The combination of heavy carbs and sugar* may leave you feeling bloated and may inhibit proper, timely elimination.
  - » Consider replacing these foods with berries, citrus, and a drizzle of honey atop of Greek yogurt. If you are dairy free, consider adding a protein source, such as nut butter, hemp seeds, or sprouted pumpkin seeds.
- *Drinking alcohol* while you're bleeding may adversely impact your hormones, which may affect the remainder of your cycle.
  - » Consider replacing it with herbal mocktails made with fresh berries, herbs, and/or bitters.
- *Caffeine* causes vasoconstriction, which slows the flow of blood and may encourage cramping.
  - » Consider replacing caffeine with dandelion or mushroom coffee. A warm cacao or golden milk latte.
- *Spicy foods* may cause digestive distress such as bloating and inflammation.
  - » Consider replacing them with foods flavored with ginger root or galangal, which have an element of heat and are also medicinal through their warming actions, which encourage healthy blood flow.

---

30 "The Importance of Maintaining a Low Omega-6/Omega-3 Ratio for Reducing the Risk of Autoimmune Diseases, Asthma, and Allergies," *The Journal of the Missouri State Medical Association*, 2021.

Moon Phase

The moon cycle begins with a new moon. In neopaganism and among others who spiritually connect with their menstrual cycle, the new moon is associated with menstruation. The darkness reflected in the moon mimics the time where the womb is in its most closed aspect. Bleeding with this phase of the moon is called a White Moon Cycle, where a person with a womb would then ovulate during the full moon. White Moon Cycles are considered to be the most common and are seen as aligned with the Mother and Nurturer archetypes. These people are thought to have an inclination to nurture creative ideas and tend to themselves and others with deep reverence. In the menstrual cycle, when one bleeds, it is time for a new cycle to begin, echoing the new moon. This moon asks us to gently prepare ourselves for what is next.

A Menstrual Phase Ritual: Create

While it may not feel authentic to be overwhelmingly productive during the menstrual phase, stepping into a creative space during this time is powerful and cathartic. (Those who experience amenorrhea, the absence of menstruation, are welcomed and encouraged to enact this ritual during a time that feels safe, held, and comfortable. The full moon or the new moon may be comforting times to choose.) For this ritual, I implore you to create something that feels as if it is a unique expression of an innermost place within.

You'll need:

- A journal and pencil/pen
- Red/pink creative tools (paint, pencils, pens, water colors, paper, fabric, thread and needle, flowers, etc.)
- A quiet, private space

Start by grounding yourself in the space you've chosen. Place a hand on your heart and a hand on your belly. Close your eyes. Focus your awareness on your breathing, noticing the pace of your inhales and exhales. Take a few moments here to steady yourself.

Imagine that your spine is like the trunk of a tree, fastening you into a grounded energy. With each inhale and exhale, visualize your spine growing roots which reach deep into the soil and through every layer of the Earth until you have hit the core.

Pause for a moment and feel the protection and healing powers of the Earth, the restorative flow it provides. Imagine a white light enveloping you, protecting you while you feel into deeper parts of yourself.

From here, tune into your womb by placing your hands over it. What messages do you hear? What colors do you see? What do you feel? What seeds of creation do you wish to plant during this more quiet, calm time in your cycle?

When you find you are satisfied with this unveiling, slowly blink your eyes open and turn to your chosen creative tools.

Create from this place. Whatever you heard, felt, saw, or experienced, create. It may be a poem. It may be splashes of color on a canvas or piece of paper. It may be a flower arrangement or an altar. When you are done, place your creation on your altar, in your workspace, or somewhere else where you will see it often.

Journal Prompts
- In what ways can you welcome more warmth into your life? How can you begin this process?
- What emotions does slowing down in life make you feel?
- What did your first cycle of bleeding feel like, emotionally, mentally, physically, and spiritually? Was it a time of rest? How do you wish it was different, if at all?
- What does feeling fully rested look like for you? Have you felt this way recently?
- What is one bit of information gleaned from the menstrual phase that you wish to bring more deeply into your life?

Follicular / Pre-Ovulatory Phase (Days 7–16)

The follicular phase technically starts the day your period begins, coinciding with the menstrual phase, and lasts until ovulation. This phase occurs as your body prepares to ovulate and release an egg, which is why this time is also referred to as the pre-ovulatory phase.

As menstruation begins, Follicle Stimulating Hormone (FSH) stimulates the development of several follicles in the ovaries, each containing an immature egg.[31] Usually, one dominant follicle continues to mature and releases increasing amounts of estrogen into the body. This rise in estrogen encourages the lining of the uterus to thicken, preparing it for a possible pregnancy.[32]

In total, the follicular phase lasts for an average of two weeks, but can last up to 21 days. This variance is precisely why it is so important to continually track your menstrual cycle through cervical fluid, position, and temperature (BBT).

As the body prepares to release an egg while also experiencing a flood of hormones, it is important to ensure you are nourishing yourself with foods and beverages that will provide dynamic support throughout these processes. Whether or not you wish for an egg to become fertilized, the body's overall health is intertwined with the health of the menstrual cycle.

As the body biologically prepares for the possibility of a pregnancy, the follicular phase echoes the season of spring, when the Earth feels full of fertile possibility. As spring rain nourishes the soil and encourages new growth, the follicular phase acts similarly within our bodies. During this time, we may

31 Carol N. Monis and Maggie Tetrokalashvili, "Menstrual Cycle Proliferative and Follicular Phase." StatPearls - NCBI Bookshelf, September 12, 2022, ncbi.nlm.nih. gov/books/NBK542229/.
32 "Follicular Phase." Cleveland Clinic, n.d., my.clevelandclinic.org/health/body/23953-follicular-phase.

feel more inspired, action-oriented, and ready to spring forward. This menstrual cycle season is an ideal time to formulate new ideas and projects.

Cervical Fluid / Position Follicular

As menstruation ends, you are not as likely to be fertile. This means there will be little to no vaginal fluid. However, if you have a shorter cycle and/or have a long bleeding time, you may still want to use backup contraception as a means of birth control, as ovulation can occur within 2 to 5 days after you stop bleeding, and sperm can survive in the vagina in the right conditions for that length of time.

The fluid present right after your period concludes will likely resemble a glue paste and be white, sticky, and crumbly when rolled between the fingers. This fluid creates a hostile environment for sperm. However, some will experience "dry" days immediately following menstruation. This is yet another great example as to why it is imperative to track your cervical fluid (CF) for many cycles to find your true pattern and to take note when shifts occur within your natural rhythm of CF, as this may alert you to shifts in the body.

As this phase progresses and more estrogen is released, cervical fluid will shift to thick, white, and maybe a bit yellowish. If yellow CF is present, there is a possibility a small amount of urine may be mixing with the CF; however, this could also be a sign of inflammation or infection and should be noted to your health care provider if other symptoms are present. The texture of CF during this part of the phase is lotion-like, and the overall feeling will be damp. When the body nears ovulation, the fluid will become more thin and cloudy.

In tandem with your cervical fluid, the cervix will become softer as the fluid becomes more wet. The closer to ovulation that you get, the higher, softer, more wet, and more open the cervix will become.

Movement

After the menstrual phase concludes, energy starts to increase. To work in tandem with your natural rhythms, slowly increase your movement activities as you embark on the follicular phase.

For the first few days after bleeding, exercises like light jogging, light weight lifting, short-distance hiking, easy vinyasa flow-style yoga, and dance classes are ideal. After those initial days, energy will start to flow with more ease. This is a great time to plan long-distance activities, high-intensity cardio, more intensive weight training, and other types of exercises that require more energy and recovery time.

Food

The follicular phase is when the body prepares the womb for the release of an egg. To do so, it needs nourishment. As hormones are released, the body works to keep them balanced and excreted from the body in a timely fashion.[33] When proper elimination doesn't occur (one healthy poop, one time a day), hormones are reabsorbed into the body through the intestinal walls. When this happens, a cascade of hormone dysregulation occurs. Therefore, during this phase, we want to eat as many nutritionally balanced foods that will support our growth and detoxification pathways.

To support the development of a maturing follicle/egg and to rejuvenate the body after bleeding, it's ideal to consume foods such as protein, healthy fats, fiber, veggies, fermented foods, nuts/seeds, and berries.

---

33 "A Prospective Study of Bowel Motility and Related Factors on Breast Cancer Risk," NIH, 2010. ncbi.nlm.nih.gov/pmc/articles/PMC2848455/.

Berries are rich in antioxidants that fight off free radicals.[34] (If free radicals aren't balanced in the body, oxidative stress occurs. This stress negatively impacts our bodies, putting them at risk for disease. It also inhibits the proper detoxification of these wastes.) As berries aren't always in season or an affordable option, consider buying bulk frozen bags, which are great for making homemade jams, including in low-sugar breakfast bakes, and adding to oatmeals and cereal.

- *Protein* provides building blocks vital to supporting the body as it prepares to release an egg. Most bodies experience the greatest nourishment and health benefits when choosing organic, pasture-raised, wild-caught, and easily digestible sources. For a healthy source of plant protein, pumpkin and flax seeds are a great choice for most as they support the healthy production of estrogen.

- *Fermented foods* are full of prebiotics and probiotics that support metabolizing and breaking down estrogen. Portion is key here. These foods should be treated as medicine. For one proper serving of ferments, drink 2 to 3 oz of kombucha, or 1 tablespoon of fermented foods. Fermented foods are one of the groups that fit into the "too much of a good thing isn't a good thing," as they can cause bloating, gas, and an upset stomach if overdone. If fermented foods aren't your thing, a good probiotic supplement may support well here, taken daily.

- *Healthy fats* modulate leptin levels, which help regulate normal ovarian function by bringing energy needed for the development of the maturing follicle, and eventually, the release of the egg during ovulation.

- *Vegetables* support the detoxification process and provide the necessary fiber needed for daily, healthy elimination.

---

34 Free radicals are unstable oxygen molecules which may create oxidative stress in the body if their levels become unbalanced.

Supportive Foods for the Late Follicular / Pre-Ovulatory Phase

- Meat/Poultry/Seafood/Protein: Wild-Caught Salmon/Tuna, Free-Range Chicken/Eggs, Tempeh, Oysters
- Vegetables: Sprouts, Broccoli, Cauliflower, Brussel Sprouts, Carrots, Sweet Potatoes, Bok Choy, Cabbage, Kale, Collard Greens, Parsley
- Fruits: Blueberries, Strawberries, Raspberries, Blackberries, Pomegranates, Apples, Avocado, Grapes, Lemons, Limes, Grapefruits
- Legumes/Nuts/Grains (Soaked & Sprouted): Flaxseed, Pumpkin Seeds, Garbanzo Beans, Almonds, Cashews, Lentils, Quinoa, Millet
- Dairy/Non-Dairy: Greek Yogurt, Grass-Fed or Raw Milk Kefir, Coconut Kefir
- Other: Sauerkraut, Kimchi, Water Kefir, Kombucha (2 to 3 oz per serving), Miso, Seaweed, Organic Nut Butters, Extra-Virgin Olive Oil, Avocado Oil, Coconut Oil, Grass-Fed Ghee/Butter

Foods to Avoid during the Follicular/Pre-Ovulatory Phase

When eating foods that do not allow for proper, timely detoxification and elimination, estrogen dominance may occur. When estrogen dominance occurs in the body, we are more likely to experience painful, uncomfortable menstruation, mood swings, depression, weight gain, migraines, and a whole slew of other symptoms that may be able to be avoided by shifting what we put into our bodies.

While what we eat isn't always the whole picture as to why we may be experiencing some of those symptoms, I would be remiss if I didn't express how much our diet interacts with our hormonal landscape.

- *Alcohol* affects how the body metabolizes estrogen and may even cause blood estrogen levels to rise. Additionally, alcohol disrupts the endocrine system, which can result in sleep disturbances, extensive stress within the body, and immune system dysregulation.[35] Therefore, alcohol isn't the most supportive thing for our bodies as they get ready for the egg to drop for ovulation.

> » Consider replacing it with CBD, which may soothe the nervous system, assist with deep sleep, and take some of the "edge" off.

- *Processed Foods* are laden with a whole number of things that are hard on our bodies. Some ingredients to look out for and generally avoid include: Artificial Flavors, Natural Flavors, Salt (Sea Salt, Himalayan Salt, or Celtic Salt is fine), Sugar (which typically means White Sugar), Colorings,[36, 37] any Gums or preservatives such as Potassium Sorbate and Sodium Benzoate.[38] Studies have shown that these ingredients inhibit many processes in the body needed for hormonal balance.[39] Simply put, these foods are hard to digest and are full of Omega-6s, which damage our cells. They also contain ingredients that confuse the brain in knowing when the body is full and usually lack much substance.

---

35 "Effects of Alcohol on the Endocrine System," NIH, 2014, ncbi.nlm.nih.gov/pmc/articles/PMC3767933/.

36 Donna McCann, Angelica Barrett, Alison Cooper, Debbie Crumpler, Lindy Dalen, Kate Grimshaw, et al, "Food Additives and Hyperactive Behaviour in 3-Year-Old and 8/9-Year-Old Children in the Community: A Randomised, Double-Blinded, Placebo-Controlled Trial," Lancet, 370(9598) (2007), 1560–1567, doi.org/10.1016/s0140-6736(07)61306-3.

37 Sarah Kobylewski and Michael F. Jacobson, "Toxicology of Food Dyes," *International Journal of Occupational and Environmental Health*, 18(3), 220–246, (2012), doi.org/10.1179/1077352512z.00000000034.

38 B. Raposa, R. Pónusz, G. Gerencsér, F. Budán, Z. Gyöngyi, A. Tibold, D. Hegyi, I. Kiss, Á. Koller, and T. Varjas, "Food Additives: Sodium Benzoate, Potassium Sorbate, Azorubine, and Tartrazine Modify the Expression of NFκB, GADD45α, and MAPK8 Genes," *Physiology International*, 103(3), 334–343, (2016), doi.org/10.1556/2060.103.2016.3.6.

39 H. Godman, "More Evidence that Ultra-Processed Foods Harm Health," Harvard Health, June 1, 2024, health.harvard.edu/nutrition/more-evidence-that-ultra-processed-foods-harm-health.

» Consider replacing these foods with: premade foods. It is surprisingly easy and quick to throw together snacks, meals, and foods for on-the-go if you schedule yourself a time to meal prep.

Moon Phase

The waxing moon and first quarter moon are deeply symbolic of the follicular phase, which like these moon phases, supplies the necessary steps for moving into the fullness experienced during ovulation. The waxing crescent moon follows the new moon, with a small sliver of light slowly pouring out from the right side of the moon. In both this moon phase and the follicular phase, this time is an invitation to foster the beginning stages of new ideas and projects and to make an intention for the unfolding cycle. The waxing crescent flows into the first quarter moon, a halfway-lit moon. The first quarter moon beckons us to commit to the theme of the cycle, whether that is a new relationship, hobby, work prospect, or idea. As we move forward with determination, more is illuminated, as is the moon, which next finds its place in the waxing gibbous stage. The moon is nearing fullness and, as such, suggests that we distill our vision into refined details, which prepare us for implementation and action, just as the follicular phase prepares the wombspace for ovulation.

A Follicular Phase Ritual: Presence

The follicular phase encourages new growth and possibility. With proper tending and intention, this growth can turn into full potential realized. Watering one's inner knowing and longings brings the fruits of tomorrow. As the saying goes, "April showers bring May flowers."

This ritual is simple and is meant to bring you into a deeper space: to consider holiness in everyday mundane activities. Active presence.

I suggest doing this ritual every morning after bleeding commences. Mornings are akin to the follicular phase, as following deep rest, one readies themselves for the day, preparing for the tasks at hand.

You'll need:

- A glass of water
- A piece of paper and a writing utensil

Pour a glass of water and go to the area where you spend your mornings. Place the glass between both hands and near your chest/heart space and close your eyes.

Recall that our bodies are made largely of water. Water nourishes our cells and is necessary for all life on Earth. Consider the holy liquid contained between your hands and bring your full awareness to what it is offering you and those you love in every moment. A prayer or spoken word of gratitude may be welcomed here.

Open your eyes and take a sip, taking note of the sensations present: the temperature, the texture, the emotional feeling. Slowly drink this glass of water, focusing only on this act.

When you are done, ask yourself: What have I watered within myself today that makes room for new growth tomorrow?

Write your answer on a piece of paper. If possible, continue to do so throughout the mornings of the remainder of the follicular phase as a reminder of how things evolve in just a matter of days.

Journal Prompts

- What new practices or activities would best support your inner growth? Do they feel within reach? If not, what are some actionable steps to assist you there?
- Do you feel inspired to rejuvenate a part of yourself spiritually, physically, mentally, or emotionally? Write down one small thing you can do to signify your desire for

this shift. How does the idea of enacting this process make you feel? Why do you think that is? Plan a time and date to move forward with this goal.

- What intention do I want to move into or focus on during this phase?
- During this follicular phase, what is my relationship with the element of water and the season of spring?
- Reflect on your last follicular phase: what has grown or shifted for you since this time?

Ovulatory Phase (Days 12–18)

Ovulation occurs when estrogen levels peak and cause an intense surge of Luteinizing Hormone (LH). Without the surge of LH, ovulation will not take place. With ovulation, the egg bursts through the follicle and is released through the ovarian wall and into the fallopian tube, where it will travel towards the uterus. The release of the egg can cause ovulation cramping, also known as mittelschmerz.

Out of all of the immature eggs, only one is released from a follicle during ovulation. However, it is possible for another egg to be released, which could result in a second pregnancy, thus creating twins. The other follicles collapse into a corpus luteum, which is a temporary organ that supports pregnancy through the release of progesterone.[40] As ovulation occurs, the follicular phase concludes.

Typically, ovulation occurs on days 12 to 18 of the cycle. However, as stated previously, every person's menstrual cycle varies. It is possible to start ovulating on day 8 of your cycle. And, it is also possible to not start ovulating for an entire month after your previous cycle has ended. (Another great reminder as to why tracking your cycle matters.)

---

40 Rebecca Oliver and Leela Sharath Pillarisetty, "Anatomy, Abdomen and Pelvis, Ovary Corpus Luteum." StatPearls - NCBI Bookshelf, January 1, 2023, ncbi.nlm. nih.gov/books/NBK539704/.

Ovulation itself occurs for 12 to 24 hours, with the phase lasting 1 to 3 days, including the day before and after ovulation. Let's break down what the previous few sentences fully mean: The fertilization of the released egg is only possible for 12 to 24 hours for the entire cycle. However, sperm can live in the vagina for up to 5 days in hospitable cervical fluid. Simply put, out of the entire cycle, there is a small window where conception can occur. If a sperm does not meet the released egg during that window of time, the egg will die.

During this phase, estrogen has peaked, and testosterone and progesterone rise, and, therefore, the summer season symbolically corresponds to the body during the ovulatory phase. This short window of the cycle offers heightened levels of energy, mood, libido, and creativity. The time is fertile, much like the sun-soaked, long days of summer. You also may notice feeling more flirty, open, receptive, and extroverted.

Cervical Fluid / Position Ovulation

As estrogen peaks in the body, there is a large increase in clear, stretchy, and egg white–like vaginal fluid, which creates conditions for sperm to live until the cervix fully opens and ovulation occurs. This is a signal that you are fertile and at or near ovulation. In total, you are fertile for only six days of any given cycle. A 1995 study showed that intercourse which occurred up to five days prior to the day of ovulation could result in a pregnancy.[41] This means, to avoid conception, it is best to avoid intercourse in this six day timeframe.

Be aware that this fluid can tend to resemble arousal fluid, but is much more stretchy. This CF is produced by the body a few days prior to and during ovulation, which may occur within

41 A. J. Wilcox, C. R. Weinberg, and D. D. Baird, "Timing of Sexual Intercourse in Relation to Ovulation— Effects on the Probability of Conception, Survival of the Pregnancy, and Sex of the Baby," *New England Journal of Medicine*, 333(23), 1517–1521, (1995), doi.org/10.1056/nejm199512073332301.

3 days before or after the last day of this type of CF appears. The absence of this fluid is important to note as it may indicate a lack of ovulation, which could hint at infertility.

During your ovulatory phase, the cervix will be high, open, wet, and soft.

Movement

Ovulation is when the body primes itself to procreate. It is providing the resources and encouragement to conceive by raising the libido, increasing energy, and gearing the body for movement.

We can channel this energy in supportive ways by taking this time to do our favorite intense workouts, if that is something that feels aligned and comfortable for our bodies. This phase can be an excellent time to plan high-energy dance classes, HIIT cardio, long-distance running, back-country backpacking, and weekend-long, activity-filled adventures, so long as they feel supportive to us.

However, our bodies' innate processes and urges will not apply to all people's wants or needs. If hormonal imbalance, chronic stress, a jam-packed busy schedule, or a run-down state is present, gentle movement such as walking, yoga, or light weight lifting should be focused on.

For ovulation cramping, try stretching practices that open your hips and relax your back.

Food

With the number of hormones coursing through the body during this phase, it is important to focus on foods that will aid in moving them out at the proper time. As you will see, the ovulatory phase has similar nutritional needs to the follicular phase, where a focus on gut health and estrogen metabolism will be highly beneficial. Light but nourishing meals typically feel best during this time. Energy is at its peak during the ovulatory phase, so prioritizing foods that sustain this energy is ideal.

- *Lean protein* will support your energy, keep you full, and will ease you more gently into the luteal phase, where energy starts to wane.
- *Fiber-rich, cruciferous, non-starchy vegetables* will aid in routine elimination and thus will assist in inhibiting estrogen dominance.
- *Quinoa, brown rice, dark, leafy greens, and cold-water fish* are densely populated with minerals and vitamins our body needs to support ovulation.
- *Wild boar, venison, bison, and elk* have become more widely available thanks to regenerative farmers who are responsibly raising and sharing these great protein sources. These proteins are less fatty, more filling, and oftentimes raised with the intention of bringing health back to the land.

Supportive Foods for the Ovulatory Phase
- Meat/Poultry/Seafood/Protein: Pasture-Raised Chicken/ Turkey/Eggs, Wild-Caught Salmon, Sprouted Tempeh, Wild Boar, Elk, Venison, Bison
- Vegetables: Spinach, Asparagus, Swiss/Rainbow Chard, Brussel Sprouts, Spirulina, Dandelion Greens, Kale, Cabbage, Turnips, Cauliflower, Bok Choy, Broccoli
- Fruits: Coconut, Figs, Dates, Apricots, Avocados, Raspberries
- Legumes/Nuts/Grains (Soaked & Sprouted): Almonds, Pecans, Quinoa, Lentils, Pistachios, Sesame Seeds
- Dairy/Non-Dairy: Coconut Kefir, Raw Milk,
- Other: Turmeric, Tahini, Bone Broth, Herb-Infused Broth

Foods to Avoid during the Ovulatory Phase
The more we can support the pathways of elimination during our entire cycle, the more we are taking care of our detoxification system so that it does not become overloaded with the surge of

hormones our bodies experience from this point of our cycle and onward. If there was any group of foods I would avoid during this time, it would be processed foods. A review of these can be found in the follicular phase section of this book.

Moon Phase

The full moon, with its open, full face, has been traditionally associated with ovulation and fertility. In neopaganism and witchcraft too, bleeding with the full moon is referred to as the Red Moon Cycle, where one will ovulate with the new moon. The Red Moon Cycle is associated with the healer archetypes: the Wise Women, the Healers, the Wisdom-Keepers, the Midwives. Spiritually, those who bleed with the Red Moon Cycle are said to have increased access to intuitive knowing, connecting with energy, sensuality, and inspiration to bring projects and ideas to fulfillment. As a typical cycle is anywhere from 19 to 32 days, give or take, a person can find themselves alternating between the White Moon and Red Moon cycles. Or, they may not bleed during either of these moon phases.

An Ovulatory Phase Ritual: Fruit

Ovulation is a creative, sensual, and energetic period during one's cycle. For this ritual, we explore these elements as the fruits of our soul's essence. Fruit contains seeds which will, in turn, create more fruit. And on and on. In the same way, creativity breeds more creativity. When we remain open, much like the cervix during this time of the menstrual cycle, we are much more readily and positively influenced by the expressions that reside within us and await our attention.

You'll need:
- Your favorite piece of fruit
- A journal and pen or pencil

Go to a comfortable area in your home or, preferably, outside. Breathe in and out of your nose to ground yourself in the moment. Place your chosen fruit in front of you. It is a visual representation of life conceived and realized into maturity. Consider the process it took for it to get to you, from all that was embedded in the soil that nourished the growing process, to the many fruits that came before it.

Say aloud: "My sensuality and creativity live within." And, take a bite of the fruit.

Write in your journal what aspects of the fruit you find beautiful (smell, taste, texture, feel). How does this remind you of your creativity and sensuality?

Say aloud: "I nourish my creativity and it nourishes me" And, take another bite of the fruit.

Write in your journal ways you tend to (or wish you did tend to) your creative dreams and process.

Say aloud: "I open myself to my creative flow and ask for its guidance" And, take another bite of the fruit.

Take a moment to close your eyes. Listen for any messages that come through. Write in your journal any images, colors, sounds, smells, or tastes that come through and feel inspiring. Do any of these things feel inspiring to your creative process?

Journal Prompts

- What is your relationship to your sensuality? How has this developed over time?
- We all have an inner creative force. How does creativity show up for you? What are you currently creating in your life?
- What experiences do you typically have or experience during ovulation?
- Are there things about your sensuality and creativity that you would like to explore, but feel intimidated by? What are they? Who do you see in your life or the public eye who has honed in on these? What was their process to tap into these things like?

Luteal Phase (Days 15–32)

As the egg is released from the follicle it was held by during ovulation, it collapses and turns into the corpus luteum. The corpus luteum will take 12 to 16 days to dissolve. If a fertilized egg is not successfully implanted, the next menstrual cycle begins. The luteal phase, on average, happens on days 15 to 32 of the cycle and ends just before the menstrual phase of the next cycle.

When the egg is released, Follicle Stimulating Hormone (FSH) and the Luteinizing Hormone (LH) drastically drops while progesterone increases. Progesterone is dispersed from the corpus luteum and will peak midway through this phase.

Progesterone has a medley of responsibilities, including:

- Preparing the uterus for a possible fertilized egg implantation
- Thickening the uterine/endometrial lining
- Stopping the body from releasing any more eggs
- Raising the basal body temperature until menstruation occurs
- Thickening cervical fluid

If a fertilized egg does not successfully implant, both estrogen and progesterone will decrease, resulting in menstruation. With the combination of those hormones dropping, serotonin and dopamine (our "feel good" hormones) tend to drop during the luteal phase as well.

The luteal phase is the autumn season of our cycle. This is the time when introspection, warming foods, and preparing for the next cycle happens. Autumn moves the hemisphere we're in into darker days, where we tend to be more introverted, focused on slowing down, and self-care. In the same way, as we wind down from ovulation towards bleeding, our energy starts to dampen and an emphasis on introspection and intuition heightens.

Cervical Fluid / Position Luteal

After ovulation, progesterone will cause cervical fluid to dry, creating a thicker, tacky fluid that is inhospitable to sperm. The closer the body gets to the menstrual phase, the drier cervical fluid will become. During this part of the cycle, the cervix will reflect similar qualities as it did in the follicular phase as it will be lower, harder, drier, and less open.

Movement

The luteal phase involves a cascade of hormones the body will need to focus on processing and eliminating. Energy naturally starts to decrease after ovulation. It may be wise to slowly taper down the intensity of movement/exercises during this time.

The closer you are to the menstrual cycle, the more you will want to conserve your energy and decrease intense exercise. Overall, supportive luteal phase movements may include strength training, pilates, and light to medium dance or aerobic classes. Studies show that consistent exercise is related to a decrease of PMS symptoms.[42]

Food

As progesterone is released in the luteal phase, the body's blood sugar becomes more sensitive. Due to this, it's important to nourish ourselves holistically during this time so that we can avoid any subsequent symptoms/mood swings. Warming foods are optimal as opposed to raw vegetables, which are more difficult to digest.

---

42 "The Effects of 8 Weeks of Regular Aerobic Exercise on the Symptoms of Premenstrual Syndrome in Non-Athlete Girls," *NIH*, 2013.

As cravings for more processed carbs are high during this time, consider eating healthier carbs like sweet potatoes, oats, wild rice, quinoa, and squash. Consuming healthy protein and fat sources as you near the menstrual phase will better prepare your body for the process of bleeding.

For deeper aid with PMS symptoms—such as general tension, difficulty sleeping, cramps, tender breasts, and headaches—magnesium-rich foods may be of aid. Symptoms such as depression, anxiety, and irritability may benefit from foods that are rich in B vitamins and Omega-3 fatty acids, such as dark, leafy greens, quinoa, wild-caught salmon, and walnuts. These foods will also encourage healthy progesterone production.

Supportive Foods for the Luteal Phase
- *Meat/Poultry/Seafood/Protein*: Wild-Caught Salmon, Tuna, Cod, Mackerel, Free Range Eggs, Pasture-Raised Turkey, Organic Tofu
- *Vegetables*: Kale, Collard Greens, Celery, Spinach, Carrots, Parsnips, Mushrooms, Squash, Bell Peppers, Chard, Kale, Spinach
- *Fruits*: Bananas, Apples, Pears, Dates, Avocado, Lemon, Lime, Grapefruit
- *Legumes/Nuts/Grains* (Soaked & Sprouted): Hempseed, Flax Seed, Aduki Beans, Garbanzo Beans, Black Beans, Sunflower Seeds, Sesame Seeds, Almonds, Wild Rice, Quinoa, Walnuts
- *Other*: Chocolate, CBD, Homemade Marshmallows (with Grass-Fed Gelatin)

Foods to Avoid during the Luteal Phase
With all of the hormones the body has to process, it would be wise to avoid processed foods as much as possible during this time. These foods tend to be high in sugar, salt, rancid oils, and

preservatives that will aggressively affect the body's ability to effectively digest all of the waste products at hand. These foods encourage bloating and excessive inflammation, which is something the body is already prone to during the later stages of the luteal phase.

In addition to avoiding processed foods, excessive cold/raw foods may not be well suited for this phase, as they are generally harder to digest and assimilate than cooked foods.

It's also worth mentioning that alcohol has a history of increasing PMS symptoms, may prevent absorption of nutrients, and may cause overall stress to the body.[43]

Moon Phase

As the full Moon concludes, it slowly moves back into darkness with the waning and third quarter moons. This movement from fullness to darkness is akin to the luteal phase, where our body prepares for the next cycle and our cervix is less open. The waning gibbous moon invites a slight absence of light on its right hand side. It asks us to let go of and release what does not support us and the ideas/projects/relationships at hand. From there, the third quarter moon comes to be—half light, half shadow. Here we find deep symbolism in preparing for a new cycle: consider both the light and the shadow. What are they showing us? Finally, before the new cycle begins, the waning crescent shines a shred of light. Spiritually, we are called to welcome the process of quieting down and resting and to let go of things that do not support the rejuvenation process the new cycle begets.

43 María Del Mar Fernández, Jurgita Saulyte, Hazel M. Inskip, and Bahi Takkouche, "Premenstrual Syndrome and Alcohol Consumption: A Systematic Review and Meta-analysis," *BMJ* Open 8, no 3 (March 2018), doi.org/10.1136/bmjopen-2017-019490.

A Luteal Phase Ritual: Calling Your Energy Back

With the luteal phase being the more introspective time of the menstrual cycle, it is an opportune time to consider all that happened and came to be during the follicular and ovulatory phases. This ritual can be done not only during the luteal phase, but also for any moment when you need restoration or an opportunity to reflect amidst stressful times in life. As we go through our days, our psychic and spiritual energy may unconsciously or consciously be held by other things, people, and/or places. A conversation, uncomfortable situation, or tough moment may leave some of your energy stuck with that person, place, or thing. Even common everyday moments can tie up our energy: work, relationships, caretaking, and projects that require our mental space. It is important that we regularly, and at least momentarily, cut off these energetic ties as they can weigh us down and keep us from fully inhabiting our bodies, making it difficult to relax our nervous systems and rest. These are all things which dampen and are "sticky" in the sense that they hold energy of yours, which tends to keep you from being fully sovereign over your life force. Calling your energy back into your body can help you find a deeper connection to what's going on internally, and thus, may help you find blocks that are keeping you from fully surrendering to rest. If the concept of "calling in your energy" is new to you, we will explore this together, in this ritual. I suggest practicing this ritual at night, before bed.

You'll need:
- Yourself
- A yoga mat
- Blanket
- Pillow or Towel

Find a comfortable space to lie down. This could be on your yoga mat, couch, floor or bed. Bring a blanket to lay over top of you and a small pillow or towel underneath your neck and knees, if needed. Get comfy.

Close your eyes and steady your breathing with long inhales and long exhales. After you feel anchored in your breath, bring awareness to how your body feels. Do a quick body scan starting with the top of the head. Place all of your energy in this space and visually direct your breath into it. What do you feel here? If any tension, pain, or uncomfortable feelings are present, imagine that your breath releases it. Continue scanning and breathing into the rest of your body, making your way towards your feet: the face, neck, shoulders, upper back, chest, upper arms, lower arms, hands, stomach, lower back, buttocks, pelvis, upper legs, knees, lower legs, feet.

As you reach your feet, take in one large cleansing breath, imagining it ripples from your head down to your toes. How does your body feel now? Do any tensions remain? What came up for you as you went through this process? Did you have a difficult time surrendering?

Next, begin the process of calling your energy back into your body. Start with the first thing that comes to mind when you think of what feels uncomfortable, stagnant, or frustrating in your life. Is this a person? A conversation? A situation? Clearly define it for yourself in your mind. As you inhale, imagine the energy you've invested and left behind lifts into the air from this mental image and makes the journey back into your body through your breath. As you do this, grant yourself the opportunity to feel the power of restoration you are offering yourself. When it feels complete, as if you've left no psychic or energetic power with this "thing," move onto the next situation, cutting off any instance which feels as if it is siphoning your energy.

As you continue to breathe with long inhales and exhales, take note of how much you feel your energy is inhabiting your body in comparison to when you began. When you have run out of specific situations that feel impending, inhale and imagine your energy in distance, unknown places floating back to you, through your nostrils. Exhale. Continue this process until you feel you are fully present with yourself. Repeat the body scan that we did at the beginning of this practice. What shifts do you notice?

Continue to lay here for a few moments, soaking in the relaxation you settle into with this practice.

Journal Prompts

- How do you prepare for a time of rest? What, if anything, stands in your way of fully resting?
- Do you regularly take time for introspection and alone time? What does this look like for you? If you don't do this, how can you start to carve out small moments for yourself?
- What do you need to relinquish from your life to better serve yourself and your ideas/projects/dreams for the next cycle?
- What lessons did you learn during this cycle? How can you grow from them and allow them to serve you?
- List ways you can prepare for the next cycle that would feel supportive. Consider choosing one and doing it by the end of the day.

Chapter Three: The Womb Life Cycle: Maiden, Mother, Crone

*M*aiden, Mother, Crone: the pages in this chapter wrote themselves with ease as I have always felt disgruntled when it came to the ways we as a culture treat the shifts that occur in the bodies of women and people with wombs.

The standard American way of welcoming ourselves into puberty, motherhood/parenthood, and the menopausal stages of life is, quite frankly, far from welcoming. In our culture, we don't have much in the way of practices and rituals to ease, support, and celebrate these transitions. But let me tell you, there are ways we can find peace within these shifts, and we'll spend this chapter examining the archetypes of Maiden, Mother, and Crone to discuss practices and rituals that celebrate all the stages of the womb life cycle—from puberty to menopause.

I ask you to consider what it would be like to live in a world where spirit, nature, and ritual are infused into every aspect of our lives. Considering that every living thing on this planet is a divine combination of nature, spirit, and ritual, it would only take a shift in the mind's eye. And with that shift? The remembrance that our bodies, each other, and our planet are worthy of our care.

This is the deep messaging behind Maiden, Mother, Crone, as this section of the book is enriched with the wisdom and presence of spirit, nature, and ritual. Things that are direct sources of empowerment, protection, and alignment of our souls and our bodies. The awareness that we are nature is forgotten by much of society. And because of that, the spirit of all things is not recognized, and our rituals have mostly melted away, aside from Hallmark holidays.

To me, it makes perfect sense that mental, spiritual, emotional, and physical imbalances blossom when we veer from the course of a life lived within the alignment of these forces, the very things we are made of and a part of.

As this is a holistic book, I wish to holistically view the issues at the core of why we don't already know this information. To start, I want to ask you to shift the messaging of what you've heard about the different phases of the womb's life cycle. I invite you to believe that these transitory periods of life as a woman don't have to be bumpy, stark, and uncomfortable. (And that sense of expected suffering is certainly the story we've been sold about having a womb.)

For as long as humans have human'd, there have been rituals, spirit-infused traditions, and plants to accompany the evolution of our bodies in each stage: Puberty, celebrated. Postpartum, a time to receive nourishment and support. And menopause, a season to bow towards the wisdom within.

In this chapter, we'll take the time to review the archetypes associated with each phase of our lives as women: Puberty through the lens of the Maiden, pregnancy through the lens of the Mother, and menopause through the lens of the Crone. These archetypes can instill within us a meaningful framework to recognize and honor these shifts.

At the end of each of the three archetypes' sections, you will find a ritual for that specific archetype. It doesn't matter what phase you are currently in—these rituals were crafted for every person to take part in at any phase. They focus on tapping into the energies we have held, currently are experiencing, or will eventually experience.

We have every right to tap into them, to find healing, and to explore what was or is yet to be. It may surprise you how much expansion you can experience with adventuring into these liminal spaces. Remember, be light and gentle with yourself when playing in this way. And, above all—have fun.

When we infuse a curious, open energy into these rituals, we release that same energy into the rest of the world, which is what will create lasting change in the dynamic we experience in society as a whole.

A Note about Other Experiences

Not all who read these words will feel aligned with the archetypes and experiences within the frameworks presented in this chapter. Know that you are welcome here. While it may not feel aligned to read the archetypal information or enact the rituals, I encourage you to consider reading the overviews on puberty, pregnancy, and menopause. We will explore more womb experiences in the following chapter.

Archetypal Overview: The Maiden

The Maiden[44] is the archetype that most embodies what most women experience from our early teens to mid-twenties. In its positive light, the Maiden's energy is empowering, confident, fertile with creativity and expansion, and full of possibility.

This archetype brings possibility and a curious nature ready to bring dreams and desires from the ethers to the surface. The Maiden nurtures these desires and interests through a willingness to explore and learn without constrictions. She creates boundaries that are respected. She feels no shame or judgment in the decisions she makes. Her sexuality is confident, free, and playful.

With these qualities, it's easy to see how The Maiden's creative force can be channeled to imbue their life with magnetism, courage, and exploration. They are paving the way for self-discovery, of their own awareness and beliefs.

---

44 Often also seen as the Virgin in varying archetypal traditions.

The Maiden is a being who is experiencing and has experienced the shift created through puberty, the first of its kind in our human experience. This evolution creates a portal of expansion, allowing for many things to come through.

By contrast, the shadow side of the Maiden can include confusion, discomfort, uncertainty, worry, and the need for acceptance. These qualities can cause naivete, the experience of being sheltered or controlled, recklessness, and disconnected embodiment.

When balanced, these shadow aspects are also the very things that light the way to unveil who you are. Still, these are things we see excessively in those who are in the Maiden chapter of their lives, due to the way our communities and structures are set up.

In an ideal world, our society would support the shift from childhood into our Maiden days in such a way that our youth would feel free to fully and rightfully embody the light -filled qualities the Maiden offers. This would look like community support of an individual's creative pursuits. Body positivity spread far and wide, a true acknowledgement that healthy bodies can come in all shapes and sizes. And sex education that focuses on teaching body and fertility awareness, allowing for folks to feel empowered by their bodies instead of scared of them.

Finding a deeper understanding of our inner Maiden creates space for us to invite others stepping into their Maiden phase to do the same.

Puberty, Explained

Puberty heralds a pivotal period in life that affects us in physiological, emotional, mental, and spiritual ways throughout our lives. For individuals with wombs, this stage signifies the onset of our reproductive years, initiating the time where we are able to conceive and carry a child.

There are three distinct physical changes that take place during puberty. They are menarche (menstruation), thelarche (breast development), and pubarche (pubic hair development). These develop over five stages, which are as follows:

- The very first stage is where nothing occurs. It is the time period where the body is considered prepubescent.
- In the second stage, thelarche commences. This typically happens between ages 7 and 13. This is the first physical sign that puberty is taking place. It is also the time when estrogen and progesterone are increased, which is what causes the breasts to develop.
- In the third stage, the body experiences pubarche. This stage usually occurs between the ages of 8 and 14. Pubic hair will appear light and sparse and increase as this stage continues. Androgens are the hormones responsible for this evolution.
- The fourth stage is where the first menstruation, menarche, occurs. The first period typically happens between the ages of 11 and 14. However, earlier menarche has been more normal in recent years. An increase in the Follicle Stimulating Hormone and the Luteinizing Hormone is what causes the first menstruation. However, the first ovulation usually will not occur for 6 to 9 months after the first period.
- The fifth, and final, stage is when puberty has concluded and physical adulthood is fully present. This can happen between the ages of 16 and 20.

Emotionally and mentally, puberty can be a difficult time for many. Emotions and behaviors become stronger and more intense. Hormones are fluctuating, weight is gained, and skin changes may be occurring.

Without nourishment and wisdom from the community, it's no wonder that many teenagers experience so much distress while experiencing puberty. If you are a person who is parenting or spending time with a person going through puberty, here are a few things that may encourage a smooth transition for this phase:

- Promote awareness of the changes that are taking place. Educational, age-appropriate materials or books may allow for a deeper understanding of what is happening to one's body. This information could be an empowering tool for a person who wants to understand why their body is changing in the ways that it is.

- Adopt a true listener's ear when large emotions and feelings arise. Staying grounded in your own energy is incredibly important when a person is experiencing frequently fluctuating moods and wants/desires that can at times be volatile and unpredictable.

- Be encouraging of who this young person is choosing to be, whether or not you understand or wish that this person would employ different hobbies or interests (unless, of course, these behaviors are dangerous to themselves or others). Ultimately, an open mind will provide an open space for that person to feel accepted and like they are allotted the expansiveness to make decisions for themselves.

A Ritual: Connecting with The Maiden

For this ritual, you'll need:

- One item each to represent (1) your emotional space, (2) your spiritual space, (3) how you felt in your physical space, and (4) how you felt supported during your Maiden years

- One item that embodies a wish you have for you in your Maiden years

- A white votive candle and something to safely burn it on

NOTE: If you have a hard time coming up with certain items that you feel represent these spaces you existed (or exist) within during your Maiden years, I encourage you to sketch something on a piece of paper so that it is a visible ensemble of items. You'll be the only one to see the sketch, so it doesn't need to be perfect.

Place the four items that represent yourself in your Maiden years in a row. In front of them, place the candle. Slightly in front of the candle, place the item that represents your wish.

When this feels complete, sit in front of this shrine without any distractions. No phones, no screens, no other people or animals in the room. If it suits you, play soft music.. Burn incense or a plant[45] that you feel connected to. Then, place your wish item in your hands and close your eyes.

Call in your guides, ancestors, angels, or higher power. Ask it or them to hold this ritual in safety and guidance.

Next, take a moment to feel the power within what your wish item represents. Visualize that power as a white, glowing light.

With each of the four items behind the candle, imagine the white light encompassing and healing each of these spaces. Take your time in doing this. Steady your breath by breathing slowly in and out of your nose. Take a moment to hold yourself in that same healing light before opening your eyes.

Then, light the candle with the intention that its light will extend the healing to the items that represent your Maiden era. Allow it to burn completely. Bury the remaining wax near your front door, or keep it in a place that you often walk near, so that its energy of light graces your days.

Journal Prompts: The Maiden

- Describe your experience with puberty. What was/is it like for you? How did/do you feel during that time?
- Where did you thrive during the ages of 11 and 18?

45 Your local apothecary or spiritual boutique may sell plant bundles for burning, such as cedar, sagebrush (not white sage, as it is overharvested and not appropriate to use unless you have grown it yourself or have purchased it from someone who did), or rosemary. Additionally, you may burn aromatic plants on a charcoal tablet used in a fire safe way.

- Where did you struggle during this time?
- What support do you wish you had?
- How can you promote a society that includes the things you wish you had?
- What parts of the Maiden archetype did you/do you embody?
- Which parts did you wish you would have embodied more?
- How do you see the intersection of the Maiden and puberty?
- Do you see ways in which we can bridge the awkward gap that exists when it comes to experiencing puberty in our society?
- What ways do you believe would have had a profound impact on inviting the positive archetypal energies of the Maiden into today's society?

Archetypal Overview: The Mother

Before diving into the Mother archetype, it's important to note that this is an archetype all women have the opportunity to embody in their lives whether or not they choose to, want to, or are able to become a mother or parent to a child of their own or one that they adopt or directly take care of. Additionally, men and non-binary people most certainly can embody the Mother.

The Mother archetype, in its positive light, embodies a feminine energy that is loving, nurturing, giving, reflective, and protective. It represents a period in life where strength, patience, and persistence are present. The Mother channels, creates, and gives life to ideas, babies, and other tangible forms. In many traditions, this archetype is associated with Mother Earth. Mother Earth takes care of and tends to the collective, not just the individual child or circumstance. Continuing from the Maiden's attributes, the Mother demands healthy boundaries and limitations. She is a person who simultaneously supports and uplifts, using her instincts to guide her.

The Mother is the archetype that a woman most commonly experiences from the mid-twenties to perimenopausal years. This person moves from the exploratory years of the Maiden into a time where creative projects, plans, babies, and ideas are nurtured and birthed. It is the pursuit of these things that is instrumental in and vital to the continuation of the holistic health of society, for the path forward is created within this timeframe. This archetype is generally respected as an embodiment that keeps the masses "fed," emotionally held, and tenderly open. Therefore, let us bring awareness to the sheer caliber of responsibility that the Mother holds.

NOTE: This book is geared toward community care, which aptly fits into the Mother's energy. Even if you do not plan on experiencing pregnancy in your life, this information is important to know and to share, as someone you know will surely be able to employ it for themselves through your assistance.

Pregnancy, Explained

When a fertilized egg is successfully implanted in the uterus, a pregnancy has occurred. Here, we will lightly discuss each phase of pregnancy, and what the human body undergoes within these time frames.

There are three phases of pregnancy, called trimesters. Some people consider there to be four, giving the postpartum experience its own timeless phase. We'll be touching on postpartum next, so for now, we will focus on the timeframe when the baby is growing inside of the womb.

First Trimester (Weeks 1–12)

The pregnant body undergoes many, many changes throughout the duration of carrying a baby. During the first trimester, these shifts may bring in symptoms, such as morning sickness, exhaustion, mood swings, tender and swollen breasts, and cravings. This is the time where the fetus develops its body structures and organs, such as its brain, stomach, intestines, and heart. Progesterone is secreted by the corpus luteum during the first ten weeks of pregnancy.[46]

Second Trimester (Weeks 13–28)
The second trimester is the middle part of the pregnancy. The symptoms discussed above typically wane as the expansion of the physical body is brought about. While energy and sleep quality are typically improved in this trimester, swollen feet, aching backs, and leg cramps may creep in during this time. Over this trimester, the baby will develop facial features, toes/fingers, and movements.

Third Trimester (Weeks 29–Birth)
In the third trimester, the baby AND the uterus are growing simultaneously, pressing up against organs even more intensely. This is why many people in this stage experience the constant need to pee, shortness of breath, and issues with sleeping. During this trimester, the baby's bones are fully forming, the lungs are developing further, and its five senses are settling in. The baby is considered full term at 39 weeks, one week prior to the due date.

Postpartum, Explained
After birth, the body is postpartum, which many refer to as the fourth trimester. Depending on who you ask, some say the postpartum period only lasts 6 to 8 weeks after the baby is born. Others say they experience this phase for years, or that a body that has given birth is forever postpartum. Many changes happen to a person after they have given birth, and those changes may include emotional and psychological aspects. While there

46 NIH, "Physiology, Progesterone," StatPearls - NCBI Bookshelf, May 1, 2023, ncbi.nlm.nih.gov/books/NBK558960/.

is a wide range of things that may be happening during the postpartum time, here are some of the most common ones:

- Breast milk develops / doesn't develop
- The perineum (the area between the vulva and rectum) may be sore, or torn, from labor
- Afterbirth cramps may be experienced as the uterus shrinks back to its normal size post pregnancy
- Lochia occurs, which is vaginal discharge that is the accumulation of the blood and tissue inside of the uterus that is expelled after birth
- Swelling of extremities, hemorrhoids, constipation, and nipple pain may be affecting the body
- Stress from having a new baby while dealing with possible exhaustion and the symptoms above may occur
- Postpartum depression or mood disorders are possible

If you have not given birth or don't plan to, I'm sure that it is now extremely clear as to why postpartum mothers need community support and care. They're undergoing a LOT while trying to juggle the task of being a new parent (or, a parent to a new baby AND other children).

A Ritual: Connecting with The Mother

For this ritual, you'll need:

- A pen or pencil
- A blank piece of paper
- Colored pencils/markers/watercolors (optional)

To begin, find a quiet space where you can be with yourself, uninterrupted. Get in a comfy seated position, or lie down. Bring in a blanket, a pillow (for under your head or knees), and light music, if needed.

Close your eyes and breathe in your nose and out of your mouth, which can be slightly open. After a few breaths, envision you are breathing all of your breath into the top of your head. As you exhale slowly, imagine your breath leaves your body through each part of you, any tension or tightness releasing with this movement—all the way to your feet.

Next, envision your breath connecting you directly to the Earth's soil. The earth, Gaia as many call her, is the embodiment of the Mother archetype in many ways. She provides us with all we have at hand: our food, our air, our homes, our water, our communities. With this in mind, feel the profound safety within imagining your breath, holding a line, an umbilical cord of sorts, to the ultimate Mother, the Earth. With every breath, visualize your breath and energy connect deeper and deeper into the Earth until you have reached its core. You'll know you have reached this spiritual space because you will feel a profound sense of being grounded. After you've arrived to this place, ask yourself, these questions:

- What do I need to nurture in my life?
- How can I connect to my creativity more deeply?
- What do I long to create?

When you feel satisfied with your answers, slowly open your eyes. Take your time arriving in the moment. When you're ready, jot down a few words or sentences that relate to your answers to the above questions.

Write these on different parts of the paper, spacing them out. Use colored pencils or pastels to depict how each word or sentence makes you feel, or the color in which you see them to be represented by. Consider that these colors may significantly nurture you and be the ones you should keep near as they are reminders of your dreams, wishes and hopes.

Journal Prompts: The Mother

- Which attributes of the Mother do you feel most connected to?
- Which do you feel you need to hone in on? Which ones do you feel disconnected from?
- Who in your life represents the Mother archetype?

- What qualities do they have that you admire?
- Which of those qualities can you see in yourself?
- How do you think you could shift your mind and life so that you embody those qualities more?
- How would you describe the Earth's motherly qualities?
- Do you have a relationship with the Earth/Mother Nature that feels deep and connected?
- Do you wish to deepen this relationship? If so, how do you envision yourself doing so?

Archetypal Overview: The Crone

How do you feel when you hear the word *Crone*? For me, it brings a sense of rich wisdom that is deeply respected: a seer whose perceptions are beyond the tangible source, a being who embodies lessons learned and implemented.

Next, how do you feel when you hear the word *menopause*? Scared? Old? Exhausted?

Recognize: Those two words are one and the same. To be in menopause is to be a Crone. To be a Crone is to have experienced or be in menopause. The more we bridge these concepts and conjoin them into one cohesive embodiment, the more power we take back our power as a collective—and the more magic and endurance we will experience as individuals. This is the path to empowerment and embodiment. And, shifting the messaging in your mind, your body, and your soul brings the collective into deeper healing.

To many, the Crone embodies the pinnacle of Source wisdom. It is gentle, but fierce; all knowing and liminal; an inward energy, while at the same time omnipresent. The word *Crone* is derived from the word *crown*, which befits the energy this archetype embodies: deep, ever-present wisdom. Do you drum up the sound of a knowing laugh when you think of this archetype? I know I do.

The Crone echoes ancient female knowledge: the matriarch that is powerful, passionate, and the culmination of living life as the Maiden and the Mother. The Crone period is a time of letting go, acceptance, and being fully in tune and aligned with the essence of que sera sera ("whatever will be, will be").

A person steps into their Crone era during perimenopause or menopause, typically around the age of fifty. This is when the body is finishing its time with the menstrual cycle, letting go of its physically fertile years, and preparing its grounds for being present with all that is.

Many times, you will hear people refer to this time with sentiments like the following: "I can't wait until I'm older and I can say whatever I want and do whatever I want." That is because the Crone answers to no one and people-pleases for nothing. They embody a beautiful, powerful, and free essence that can't quite be held onto.

My wish is that the power and respect the Crone demands is instilled into our culture, more and more. I believe our society will be enriched with the wisdom we need most when we re-learn how to tend to, receive, and support our Crones. After all, it is shown that community and support during this time has proven to lessen the severity of menopausal symptoms, nodding to the notion that shifting the stories and the way we view this time in our lives really, truly matters.[47]

Menopause, Explained

When the body starts winding down its fertile years, the cycle of menopause has begun. Three phases occur during this transition, which include perimenopause, menopause, and post-menopause.

---

47 "Role of Social Support in Reducing the Severity of Menopausal Symptoms among Women Living in Rural Mysuru, Karnataka: An Analytical Cross-sectional Study," *Journal of Mid-Life Health*, 2024.

Perimenopause is the 3 to 8 year period where hormones start to decline and shift. The ovaries slowly decrease their function. Less estrogen is produced, causing ovulation to be irregular and eventually stop altogether. Thus, the menstrual cycle may include a longer cycle or stop and start with no predictability. This may be accompanied by hot flashes, vaginal dryness, sleep issues, and mood changes. Perimenopause can begin as early as the late thirties or forties.

Menopause officially occurs when 12 months have passed since the last bleed. Do note that this does not include times where one is pregnant, breastfeeding, or on medication that may interfere with ovulation. Events that may cause early menopause include a person having a hysterectomy (the removal of the uterus), an oophorectomy (where the ovaries are removed), or underactive/inactive ovaries due to treatments such as radiation or chemotherapy. Menopause is communication that the body has stopped producing eggs and estrogen is significantly decreased. Symptoms of menopause include night sweats, insomnia, a general dry feeling to tissue states, change in libido, hair loss/thinning, weight gain, and heart palpitations. Not all people will experience these symptoms, and some people will not experience any symptoms.

Post-menopause is the time after menopause. Symptoms experienced in perimenopause and menopause may continue or decrease. The body may continue to change. During this time, it is important that healthy lifestyle habits are prioritized.

A Ritual: Connecting with the Crone

For this ritual, you'll need:

- A flower, heirloom, or relic to represent the past
- A journal and pen and paper (optional)

Find a comfortable, private space and get cozy. Place your flower, heirloom, or relic in front of you. If possible, put it at eye level so that you can easily observe it. Gaze into the object, noting every crevice, shade, color, and feature it holds.

Next, ask these questions (aloud, if possible) and contemplate their answers. Take your time with this. Write down your answers if you feel called to do so.

- What came before you?
- Who created you? And how?
- What had to be learned to create you?
- Who was the original source of this wisdom?

Once you feel the magnitude of this final answer, close your eyes and breathe in and out of your nose, focusing on its energy. The Crone's energy is inevitably and intrinsically a part of this energy and object, for there is no thing or no one who is not touched by the wisdom of the Crone. Feel the power that was involved in bringing this object to you. Speculate at the accumulation of wisdom required to get this thing to the point where it is now. Ask yourself where you can embody this same energy in your life, and what it may do for you.

When you are finished, feel free to journal or set an intention of how you can apply what you've discovered into your life.

Journal Prompts: The Crone

- How have you traditionally viewed menopause?
- Have your views on menopause changed after reading this chapter?
- Do you see the ways in which menopause can be enriched by the presence of the Crone's archetypal energy?
- Who are the people in your life or that you know of who embody the Crone?
- Which of them do you admire? And why do you think that is?
- Do you now feel more readily suited to experience menopause?

Chapter Four: Other Womb Experiences

*T*here are too many of us who suffer in silence and alone when it comes to the chronic pains/side effects of irregular menstruation, the experience of pregnancy loss, and the emotional toll that being a woman in society entails. There are a wide variety of womb experiences one may have that don't fit as neatly into the Maiden/Mother/Crone archetypes. While it is impossible for me to cover all womb experiences one may have, I've worked hard to provide an overview of some of the most common ones.

For this chapter, if you wish to integrate a womb experience with your practice as a witch, explore the "Connect Deeper" options offered with each situation reviewed.

Painful Periods, Dysmenorrhea

Dysmenorrhea, the pain that is associated with menstrual cramps, is thought to occur when prostaglandins (compounds in the uterine tissues that act like hormones) cause the uterus to contract.

This pain may sometimes be accompanied by diarrhea, constipation, vomiting, and fatigue. These contractions, if strong enough, can press against blood vessels in the area, thus preventing normal blood flow and oxygen to the muscle, which then causes pain.

Connect Deeper: When experiencing pain, we are likely to take in frantic, shallow, and fast-paced breaths. This can extend our nervous system into a frazzled state, which can further exacerbate our symptoms. Breathwork, also known as pranayama in the yogic tradition, is an ancient practice which utilizes the breath to direct a calming effect on the nervous system.

Prior to the menstrual phase, you can use the following steps for this simple breathwork practice to calm your mind and body during painful symptoms.

Step 1: Sitting upwards, close your eyes and take a long breath through your nose into your belly. Do so to the count of 4.

Step 2: Exhale slowly through your nose. Again, to the count of 4.

Step 3: Repeat several times, or until you feel your energy start to settle.

PMS and PMDD

You've most certainly heard of PMS, which is short for premenstrual syndrome. Maybe you've even been the victim of someone murmuring not-so-silently under their breath, "Watch out—they're PMSing." As it happens, the majority of menstruating people will experience PMS at some point in their lives. It is THAT common of an experience. The main actors in PMS symptoms are imbalances in sex hormones, stress hormones, and neurotransmitters.

PMS may be exacerbated by dietary factors, stressful events, thyroid issues, and mineral deficiencies. These symptoms typically occur around one week prior to the start of menstruation, but may occur earlier for some.

Premenstrual syndrome encompasses over 150 different symptoms. However, common signs and symptoms include bloating, fatigue, mood swings, depression, irritability, breast tenderness, food cravings, and skin issues. These symptoms are signals that the body may be in need of additional supplementation, diet tweaks, more movement, rest, and/or stress reduction.

PMDD (Premenstrual Dysphoric Disorder) is a more severe form of PMS that has both physical and emotional symptoms[48] that tend to be more drastic. Mood swings, anxiety, anger, and depression are common emotional symptoms present with PMDD. Physically, acne, muscle spasms, hot flashes, and nausea may arise.[49]

Connect Deeper: Symptoms are communications from the depths of ourselves. They can be spiritual, physiological, mental, and/or emotional in nature. To seek a pathway that integrates these messages, our needs must be prioritized. If you are experiencing PMS symptoms, consider the following: What are your needs right now? What would it feel like to compassionately honor what you're experiencing? Create a simple mantra, or invocation, that represents you getting your specific needs met. Chant it aloud or in your head several times. Then, call on this mantra when you are in need of its power.

Endometriosis

Endometriosis is a condition that occurs when tissue that is similar to the tissue found in the uterus, called endometrium, grows outside of the womb and onto different parts of the body. This tissue commonly grows outside of the uterus onto the fallopian tubes, ovaries, and tissues surrounding the uterus.

However, endometrium tissue can also grow on the bladder, rectum, vagina, and bowels, among other places. It is theorized that endometriosis affects 1 in 10 women in the US, although it is extremely difficult to diagnose without surgery, leading

---

48 Mayo Clinic, "Premenstrual Dysphoric Disorder: Different From PMS?", January 19, 2024, mayoclinic.org/diseases-conditions/premenstrual-syndrome/expert-answers/pmdd/faq-20058315#:~:text=Answer%20From%20Tatnai%20Burnett%2C%20M.D.

49 Johns Hopkins Medicine, "Premenstrual Dysphoric Disorder (PMDD)," April 26, 2024, hopkinsmedicine.org/health/conditions-and-diseases/premenstrual-dysphoric-disorder-pmdd.

many people to remain in the dark about whether or not they technically have endometriosis.

Chronic pain, infertility, bleeding or spotting in between menstruation, and digestive system problems are the main symptoms of endometriosis. Endometriosis growths may bleed and become inflamed similar to uterine linings during menstruation, which can cause extreme pain as the blood cannot exit the body as readily.

There is no known, definitive cause of endometriosis. Factors such as estrogen dominance, autoimmune disorders, genetic predisposition, and certain cancers are commonly found in bodies with endometriosis. There is no cure for endometriosis, but there are options available to manage symptoms and improve quality of life.

Connect Deeper: Endo comes from the Greek word endon, meaning "in, within, internal." I speak as someone who experiences endometriosis: Within a person who experiences this condition is a deep well of strength. Consider where you feel internally connected in a way that brings light to your being. How does this connection create stores of power within? Find a small object to represent this source. Place it between your hands and infuse it with prayer, meditation, spoken word, or song. After completing this ritual, you might find that your chosen object may be a nice addition to your altar or may be a comforting item to hold during flare-ups.

PCOS

Polycystic Ovarian Syndrome, or PCOS, is thought to affect 10 to 15 percent of women in their child-bearing years. The jury is still out on the definitive cause of PCOS, but there are several scientific theories about why folks have this condition.

Generally, there is some sort of hormonal imbalance, low-grade inflammation, and/or insulin resistance present. Because of these possible underlying factors, it is important to take a clinical diagnosis of PCOS seriously, as insulin resistance is the precursor to diabetes, heart disease, and stroke. While genetic factors do play a role in a person's risk of having PCOS, it is worth noting that lifestyle habits—such as a balanced diet, consistent sleep schedule, effective stress management, and regular physical activity—may also significantly impact its development and management.

The major symptoms present in an individual with PCOS include acne, abnormal hair growth, abnormal weight gain, infertility or irregular ovulation, hair thinning/loss, and some psychological effects such as depression and anxiety.

While weight gain or higher body weight is associated with PCOS, it is important to note that professional, extremely fit athletes are diagnosed with this condition as well. Over-exercising is a stressor, and it's something that should be avoided if it is aggravating the body. However, balanced exercise is an important option to consider with PCOS, as lean muscle is a factor that helps curb and control blood sugar imbalances,[50] which is why weight loss is what is typically recommended when addressing PCOS.

Connect Deeper: Dealing with health grievances of any kind can bring in the feeling of loss of control. As mentioned previously in this book, words are spells that direct energy. To direct is to take control. For this spell, make a list of things you have control over and choose in your life. Think about listing a variety of things—a mixture of surface- and deeper-level statements.

Examples:

I choose to listen to music that makes me feel good.

I choose to keep friends close that support me.

I choose to read books that inspire me.

50 "Increasing muscle mass to improve metabolism." *Adipocyte*, 2013.

I choose to love myself unconditionally.

I choose to welcome my shadow and integrate its lessons.

I choose to allow myself to feel my emotions deeply.

Say them aloud from the heart.

Fibroids

Fibroids are solid, defined muscle and connective tissue growths that exist on the uterus. They are noncancerous (benign) growths that can cause discomfort and infertility and are one of the main causes of premenopausal hysterectomies. It is estimated that a whopping 70 to 80 percent of women in the U.S. will develop fibroids in their lifetime. However, not all of these cases will cause debilitating issues or discomfort.

There are three different kinds of fibroids.

- Subserosal fibroids, which grow on the outer edges of the uterus and sometimes push out of that area into the pelvis. These are the most common kinds of fibroids
- Intramural fibroids, which develop in the muscular walls of the uterus.
- Submucosal fibroids, which grow into the uterine cavity and are the least common.

Excess estrogen causes fibroids to grow. Experiencing estrogen dominance for several decades may lead to the development of fibroids, which is why these are mostly experienced by folks in their forties. While there is no known cause of fibroids, the populations most at risk for developing them include people over the age of 30, folks with higher body weight to body fat proportions, those experiencing estrogen dominance, those with a family history of fibroids, and Black women/people with wombs.

Stress, dietary factors, Vitamin D deficiency, excess plastic exposure, racial discrimination, and trauma are all factors that contribute to increasing your likelihood of developing fibroids.

After menopause, the risk for developing severe issues with fibroids is highly decreased, as estrogen has also decreased.

Symptoms of fibroids can range from a discomfort level of "Maybe I have fibroids?" to "Holy shit, this is ruining my life," which is often why a large percentage of people choose to have a hysterectomy. These symptoms include:

- Heavy, long menstruation
- Severe menstrual cramps
- Constipation
- Abdominal cramps
- Frequent or difficulty with urination
- Abnormal uterine bleeding
- Infertility
- Pain during intercourse

Connect Deeper: Our wombs are sources of creativity, sensuality, and deep, intuitive wisdom. Without the ability or support to express these innate desires, our overall energy becomes stagnant and suppressed and stress is likely lurking around the corner. Name one of your unfulfilled deepest desires. Give it an offering. Write a poem, sketch a drawing, bring forth a dance, sing a song. This act signals to the universe you are ready to bring it to life: a release and an opening. This is an alchemical way of turning something deep within you into a source of magick. Relate this to your physical body. How can this release offer your womb a similar experience?

Ovarian Cysts

Ovarian cysts are fluid-filled sacs typically on or near the ovaries. Cysts commonly appear from the onset of menarche until the beginning of menopause and are thought to form during ovulation. They often disappear without any symptoms, but also have the capacity to cause issues and deep pain when erupting.

The two most common types of ovarian cysts are:

- Follicle cysts: Formed when the follicles meant to release a mature egg do not break open, causing the follicle to grow into a cyst.
- Corpus luteum cysts: When the follicle does release the egg, it turns into the corpus luteum. When the corpus luteum does not shrink, as it normally does, it reseals itself and turns into a corpus luteum cyst. These are known to possibly grow up to four inches and may cause twisting of the ovaries, leading to pain.

Cysts are theorized to be caused by hormonal issues or medications that promote ovulation. Symptoms include feeling pressure in the abdomen, breast tenderness, pain during sex, unexplained weight gain, and a frequent urge to urinate.

Connect Deeper: Sacred spiritual texts are scattered with stories where healing occurs with the use of touch and hand movements. In today's society, this is often offered as therapeutic touch, reiki, or healing touch. While training in this healing modality will enhance our ability and understanding of this therapy, we are absolutely capable of providing ourselves with healing touch independently. To do so, use the following steps:

Step 1: Sitting upright or lying down, place both of your hands on your wombspace, just below the belly button.

Step 2: Breathing in and out slowly and steadily, imagine a white light enveloping your hands. Into this light, send thoughts of love, compassion, openness, courage, and peace.

Step 3: As you continue to breathe, imagine this light penetrating through your skin into your wombspace, filling it with this intentionally infused light.

Amenorrhea

The absence of menstruation during a person's reproductive years is called amenorrhea. This can occur in both the short and long term, happening for the span of a minimum of three cycles and extending over years. Causes of amenorrhea may include use of birth control pills/IUD, menopause, pregnancy, breastfeeding, delayed puberty, weight loss, hormone disruption, tumors, PCOS, hypothalamic amenorrhea, hyperprolactinemia, and Cushing syndrome.[51]

While it is estimated only 1 percent of women in the U.S. experience amenorrhea, there has been increasing promotion of birth control methods that cause a person's period to cease, specifically hormonal birth control and IUDs. It is important to know about the risks involved in choosing these options as oftentimes the long-term implications are not divulged by our health practitioners. The risks of long-term amenorrhea include increased risk of hip and wrist fracture, osteoporosis, fertility issues, cardiovascular disease (related to exercise-induced secondary amenorrhea), and pelvic pain.[52, 53, 54]

Connect Deeper: Cosmic voids are dark spaces, much like our wombs. As above, so below. This nothingness, as it is called, is spiritually seen as the gateway to manifestation. Whether we have a monthly bleed or not, we can harness the magick held within our wombs. Here, we can bring to life that which is inspired within the deepest parts of ourselves. What have you willed into existence in this life? How has it brought joy to yourself, to those you love, to strangers? Find a way to exalt this in the material realms: through an outfit, rearranging your

51 Gul Nawaz, Alan D. Rogol, and Suzanne M. Jenkins, "Amenorrhea," StatPearls - NCBI Bookshelf, February 25, 2024. ncbi.nlm.nih.gov/books/NBK482168/.

52 Mayo Clinic, "Amenorrhea - Symptoms and Causes - Mayo Clinic," February 9, 2023, mayoclinic.org/diseases-conditions/amenorrhea/symptoms-causes/syc-20369299.

53 Catherine M. Gordon and Lawrence M. Nelson, "Amenorrhea and Bone Health in Adolescents and Young Women," *Current Opinion in Obstetrics & Gynecology/ Current Opinion in Obstetrics & Gynecology, With Evaluated MEDLINE* 15, no 5 (October 1, 2003): 377–84, doi.org/10.1097/00001703-200310000-00005.

54 Nicole L. Tegg, Caitlynd Myburgh, Megan Kennedy, and Colleen M. Norris, "Impact of Secondary Amenorrhea on Cardiovascular Disease Risk in Physically Active Women: A Systematic Review Protocol," *JBI Evidence Synthesis*, August 2, 2023, doi.org/10.11124/jbies-23-00047.

altar, making a flower arrangement with wild botanicals, putting paint to canvas, or through singing a song that is reminiscent of what you've brought into this life.

Pregnancy Loss

Whether we know it or not, we all know someone who has experienced a pregnancy loss or abortion. It is that common of an occurrence. It is estimated that 1 in 4 pregnancies will end in miscarriage[55] and in 2022, 1 in every 72 pregnancies ended in stillbirth.[56] These are staggering numbers, especially when considering the aftermath and emotional toll this experience has on a body and mind. There isn't a deep presence of care in our society for the people who experience miscarriage, ectopic pregnancy, abortion, or stillbirth. And to top it off, I've found through personal experience, as well as anecdotal experiences others have shared with me, that people who experience pregnancy loss or choose to release their pregnancy are oftentimes left in the dark when it comes to what happened and will happen to their bodies in the coming days and weeks. This is a heartbreaking and dangerous failure of our health practitioners and educational systems.

Body literacy is incredibly important for those who are engaging in sex which has the possibility of resulting in a pregnancy. This knowledge can save a life. It can relax our mental spaces, even if slightly, because we will have a better idea of what is happening and what has happened to our bodies. It can also allow us to nurture and care for another who is experiencing this profoundly difficult experience. We will next

55 PubMed, "Miscarriage (Archived)," January 1, 2024, pubmed.ncbi.nlm. nih.gov/30422585/#:~:text=The%20American%20College%20of%20 Obstetricians,10%25%20of%20clinically%20recognized%20pregnancies.
56 UNICEF, "Stillbirths and Stillbirth Rates - UNICEF DATA," May 6, 2024, data. unicef.org/topic/child-survival/stillbirths/#:~:text=Around%201.9%20million%20 stillbirths%20%E2%80%93%20babies,stillbirths%20per%201%2C000%20total%20 births.

be reviewing miscarriage, abortion, ectopic pregnancy, molar pregnancy, and stillbirth in this section.

A word on semantics: Many people are surprised to find out the medical terminology for miscarriage typically is labeled by practitioners and in medical files as a spontaneous, missed, incomplete, or complete abortion. The government, our media, and the general public have certainly demonized the word *abortion* and its complete definition and action. Britannica defines abortion as, "the expulsion of a fetus from the uterus before it has reached the stage of viability."[57] This can involve choice or happen, as medically defined, spontaneously. Like the word *witch*, the word *abortion* needs reclaimed. Abortion is a natural process and one women have experienced and performed for ourselves for as long as we have experienced pregnancy.

Miscarriage

Miscarriage is the term for pregnancy loss in the first 20 weeks of pregnancy. For many of these miscarriages, the cause is unknown, with many of them occurring in the first trimester. Some warning signs of miscarriage include mild to severe back pain; uterine cramping/contractions; vaginal bleeding, which can be normal in early pregnancy but should be closely monitored; passing blood clots; and dizziness and fever.

There are different types of miscarriages, which include incomplete, complete, threatened, inevitable, and missed miscarriages, as well as chemical pregnancy and blighted ovum. Let's discuss the differences between these.

An *incomplete miscarriage*, also called an *incomplete abortion*, occurs when not all of the pregnancy tissue is passed. One can expect heavy vaginal bleeding and strong uterine cramps. It is important to receive a checkup with a midwife or

---

57 The Editors of Encyclopaedia Britannica, "Abortion | Definition, Procedure, Laws, & Facts," Encyclopedia Britannica, May 17, 2024, britannica.com/science/abortion-pregnancy.

physician to ensure a person is not experiencing an incomplete miscarriage, as this type of miscarriage has the possibility of resulting in dilation and curettage, a minor surgical procedure. This procedure, known as a D&C, will remove any leftover pregnancy tissue.

A *complete miscarriage* may also be called a *complete abortion*. This type of miscarriage fully expels pregnancy tissue from the uterus. It is common for vaginal bleeding to continue for a few days, accompanied by contractions or strong cramps as the uterus is emptying.

Vaginal bleeding during the first 20 weeks of pregnancy is considered a *threatened miscarriage*. Other symptoms that arise with threatened miscarriages include lower back and abdominal pain. Here the cervix will remain closed. Half of threatened miscarriages end in a live birth.

When one experiences light, unexplained vaginal bleeding and cramping during the early phase of pregnancy, this is called an *inevitable miscarriage*. A threatened miscarriage may develop into an inevitable miscarriage if the cervix dilates. Once tissue passes through the cervical canal, it becomes an incomplete miscarriage, and eventually a complete miscarriage.

A *missed miscarriage*, also known as a *missed abortion*, occurs when the fertilized egg implants but does not develop. However, in this type of miscarriage, the body does not expel the pregnancy. Symptoms include experiencing brown discharge and lower back or abdominal cramping. Oftentimes, many do not know that the fetus has died. This is typically discovered through a regular ultrasound.

A *chemical pregnancy* occurs before one may even be able to know they are pregnant, within the first five weeks of pregnancy. In this type of miscarriage, the fertilized egg does not develop. This often occurs due to chromosomal abnormalities. The embryo may possibly implant before it stops developing. Most people who experience a chemical pregnancy do not know that they are miscarrying, as it usually occurs during one's period.

Similar to a chemical pregnancy, a *blighted ovum* occurs when an embryo attaches to the uterus, but does not develop. This occurs very early in the pregnancy, in the first five weeks.

Safety Note: For any type of miscarriage, a checkup is highly recommended to ensure that a person's body has completed the miscarriage and that no pregnancy tissue remains in the uterus.

Connect Deeper: Isis, Artemis, Freyja, Durga, Hera: ancient, timeless deities who are protectors of women; symbols of strength, motherhood, and childbirth; and associated with healing. Choose a deity from this list, or a figure of women/childbirth that you connect with, and spend some time bridging a relationship with them. Steep yourself in their mythology, connect with their energy, make them an offering on your altar, and explore where they can assist you in your healing process from the experience of a miscarriage.

Abortion

Colloquially, abortion is often described as the decision to release a pregnancy. However, this oversimplification ignores those who choose to get pregnant and find it is medically necessary to have an abortion. There are many complex reasons why one may choose or medically need to release their pregnancy, and each is specific to the individual. A survey from the Guttmacher Institute found that one in four women in America will have an abortion by age 45.[58]

There are two primary medical options for abortion: an in-clinic procedure and a medication (pill) option. The method of receiving an abortion varies from state to state and is something that is, as of writing this book, constantly changing. Some states

---

58 Guttmacher Institute, "One in Four US Women Expected to Have an Abortion in Their Lifetime," April 29, 2024, guttmacher.org/news-release/2024/one-four-us-women-expected-have-abortion-their-lifetime.

require that you wait 24 hours after your initial appointment before you can get the abortion, while some allow it to happen the same day. With this in mind, I highly suggest you familiarize yourself with your state's abortion laws, whether or not you are currently or ever engaging in sex that could result in a pregnancy. While, at the time of writing this, medical abortion access in the U.S. has or is being threatened in various states, these procedures and medications are incredibly safe options that save lives by being made accessible.[59]

For in-clinic abortions, there are typically two options: suction/aspiration abortion and a Dilation and Evacuation (D&E) abortion. The suction/aspiration abortion may be provided until 14 to 16 weeks from the last menstruation. This procedure usually takes 5 to 10 minutes. Numbing or pain medication is offered, the cervix is dilated, and the pregnancy tissue is removed with an aspirator or suction.

A D&E is the common procedure for those who have an abortion later than 14 to 16 weeks. This procedure takes longer than the suction/aspiration procedure, lasting around 15 to 30 minutes. However, because these pregnancies are more advanced, they may require a two-day procedure so that the cervix may gradually dilate. The procedure may involve some form of sedation or pain medication, then the pregnancy is removed with suction and instruments by the provider.

While the procedures themselves do not take an excessive amount of time, do keep in mind that the appointment in total will take longer and vary from clinic to clinic. As with most other pregnancy releases, bleeding and cramping are normal things to experience and will accompany an in-clinic abortion.

Medication abortion, also known as the abortion pills, are available to those who are early in their pregnancy, typically

59 "The Safety and Quality of Abortion Care in the United States," n.d., ncbi.nlm. nih.gov/books/NBK507236/.

below 10 to 11 weeks. Two different types of pills, mifepristone and misoprostol, are used in medication abortion. Mifepristone is taken first and stops progesterone from being released into the body, which causes the pregnancy to cease developmentally. Next, misoprostol is taken to empty the uterus of pregnancy tissue, which should occur within 24 hours of taking the pill. Heavy cramping, bleeding, nausea, and fatigue are common symptoms that occur with the pill. Commonly, clinics will schedule a follow-up appointment one to two weeks after to ensure all of the pregnancy tissue has passed. Medication abortions have an efficacy to terminate pregnancy 98 percent of the time.[60]

Safety Note: While complications with early medical abortions are a rare occurrence, there are serious symptoms to be aware of. According to AbortionPillInfo.org, if someone is experiencing any of these, it is important to seek immediate medical attention:

- bleeding through more than 2 maxi pads an hour for more than 2 hours
- experiencing severe pain, which is not relieved with pain-killers, for more than 2 to 3 days
- fever that reaches 100 degrees F for more than 24 hours, or a fever that reaches 102 degrees F at any point[61]
- Abnormal vaginal discharge that gives off an unpleasant smell and/or is green/yellow in color[62]

Connect Deeper: Not all folks experience their abortion in spiritual or emotional ways and may view their abortion as simply a medical procedure that was needed. Some will endure a grieving process that lasts weeks, months, or years, and some will require deeper spiritual navigation. I invite you to allow

---

60 "Abortion in Clinic: What to Expect - National Abortion Federation, June 4, 2024, prochoice.org/patients/abortion-what-to-expect/.
61 WomenHelp SASS, "How to Use Abortion Pills," n.d., abortionpillinfo.org/en/using-abortion-pills-for-safe-abortion-usa.
62 "How to Use Abortion Pills."

room for whatever embodiment this experience was for you. This is your deep knowing.

Meditation allows us to bring focus within, offering us an opportunity to clarify, heal, and focus on a specific subject or issue.

Find a comfortable seated position in a calm, quiet environment. Close your eyes and steady your breath with even inhales and exhales through the belly. Allow the deep knowing within to arise. Focus on its energy. There is no need to push or dig. You may see colors, hear messages, or find a mantra that comes to the surface. Allow these things to come and go, surrendering to the moment and freeing yourself from the impulse to control the experience. Stay here for whatever amount of time feels supportive. Consider repeating this process in the days, weeks, months, or years that follow.

Ectopic Pregnancy

Ectopic pregnancy occurs when a fertilized egg implants outside of the uterus, which can happen in the fallopian tube, ovary, abdomen, or cervix. This type of pregnancy is dangerous, as when left untreated, it can result in death due to hemorrhaging. One in every 100 pregnancies is an ectopic pregnancy. As the pregnancy grows, it may cause the fallopian tube to rupture and cause internal bleeding to occur. Ectopic pregnancies occur for a medley of reasons that include scarring due to previous infection or surgery, endometriosis, hormonal factors, birth defects, and medical conditions that affect the shape of the reproductive organs.

Signs and symptoms of an ectopic pregnancy include light bleeding, extreme abdominal pain, dizziness/weakness, pain on one side of the body, and upset stomach and/or diarrhea. These symptoms are often accompanied by a positive pregnancy test as they do produce the hormone necessary for a positive pregnancy test, hCG.

These pregnancies are not viable and CANNOT be reimplanted. They must be removed, whether through surgery or a pill.

The surgery that accompanies ectopic pregnancy will most commonly be a salpingostomy or a salpingectomy, which are laparoscopic surgeries.

In a salpingostomy, the pregnancy is removed and the fallopian tube remains. With a salpingectomy, both the pregnancy and the tube are removed, as the tube is irreparably damaged or has ruptured.

The medication offered to terminate an early ectopic pregnancy where unstable bleeding isn't present is called methotrexate, which is delivered in the form of an injection or a pill. This medication terminates the pregnancy by stopping cell proliferation and dissolving the cells that do exist.

Connect Deeper: Whether the body experiences surgery or receives an injection or pill that results in the release of a pregnancy, the experience generally is chaotic and ungrounding to our biology. Grounding our energy through planting our feet or hands directly on the Earth's surface is an electrically conductive process. This act transfers the Earth's free electrons into our bodies with this direct contact.[63] These electrons have been shown in studies to bring forth anti-inflammatory, wound healing, and positive immune response reactions.[64]

Go outside. Find a place that feels comfortable and position your bare feet onto the Earth or place your hands onto a tree, which enacts the same process. Feel yourself harnessing the Earth's energy and allow it to comb over your nervous system

63 G. Chevalier,S. T. Sinatra, J. L. Oschman, K. Sokal, and P. Sokal, "Earthing: Health Implications of Reconnecting the Human Body to the Earth's Surface Electrons. *Journal of Environmental and Public Health*, 1–8, (2012), doi. org/10.1155/2012/291541

64 "The Effects of Grounding (Earthing) on Inflammation, the Immune Response, Wound Healing, and Prevention and Treatment of Chronic Inflammatory and Autoimmune Diseases," *Journal of Inflammation Research*, 2015.

and body. Stay with this energetic exchange for as long as you need. Return to this practice as often as needed.

Molar Pregnancy

A molar pregnancy is rare, affecting only 1 in 100 pregnancies. This type of pregnancy is the result of an abnormal growth of cells that normally grow in the placenta due to an atypical fertilized egg, resulting in fluid-filled cysts and nearly no fetal tissue growth. Molar pregnancies can have extreme issues, which include serious nausea and vomiting; pelvic pressure, inflammation, and pain; hyperthyroidism; preeclampsia; and ovarian cysts.

There are two types of molar pregnancy, complete and partial. With a complete molar pregnancy, the egg contains only the sperm's genetic material, duplicating the chromosomes of the sperm. In a partial molar pregnancy, the egg's chromosomes are present with two sets of the sperm's chromosomal material. A D&C is usually performed for a molar pregnancy. However, molar pregnancy tissue may continue to grow, which is sometimes treated with chemotherapy.

Those who have had previous molar pregnancies or are over the age of 35 are more likely to experience a molar pregnancy in the future.

Connect Deeper: All of life on Earth is present thanks to all of the elements: earth, wind, fire, water, spirit. Of these elements, our bodies are made up largely of water. Choose a plant or tree that is inside of or surrounds your home. One that you feel connected to or wish to develop a connection to. Fill up a cup of water and hold it between your hands. Feel its offering of nourishment. Consider how connected this element is to our every breath. Recognize the life force that it offers. Pray into these waters, offering words which feel healing for your pregnancy loss. Mindfully take that water to your plant or tree of choice and offer its contents to its soil. With this act of reciprocity, you nourish yourself and your own soils. Thank the plant. Thank yourself. Make this a weekly ritual for as long as it feels accessible and nourishing.

Stillbirth

A stillbirth occurs before or during delivery. In the U.S., this is the way a pregnancy loss is termed when the baby is lost after 20 weeks of gestation. It is estimated that less than 1 percent of pregnancies will result in a late-term miscarriage or stillbirth. While two-thirds of stillbirths will result in a medical explanation, the remainder will remain unexplained, according to the Cleveland Clinic.

Common explained causes of stillbirth include issues with the placenta and umbilical cord, infections, birth defects, high blood pressure, and lifestyle factors, such as drug use, drinking, and tobacco use. Those who have extra body weight or are underweight, have a preexisting condition, are having multiple births, have poor prenatal care, or are over the age of 35 are at a greater risk for stillbirth.[65, 66, 67]

For those who experience a stillbirth prior to delivery, or if it is anticipated, labor is often induced. However, natural labor may be an option as well, depending on the situation. After birth, bleeding may occur for 5 to 10 days and possibly longer. If blood clots are larger than a grape, or if bleeding soaks one pad an hour, seeking medical attention is vital.

In addition to bleeding, breast tenderness and possible milk leakage may occur. The perineum and vagina may be sore

65 "The Impact of Isolated Obesity Compared with Obesity and Other Risk Factors on Risk of Stillbirth: A Retrospective Cohort Study," CMAJ, 2024, ncbi.nlm.nih.gov/pmc/articles/PMC10911866/.

66 Ruofan Yao, Bo Y. Park, Sarah E. Foster, and Aaron B. Caughey, "The Association Between Gestational Weight Gain and Risk of Stillbirth: A Population-Based Cohort Study." *Annals of Epidemiology* 27, no 10 (October 1, 2017): 638-644.e1, doi.org/10.1016/j.annepidem.2017.09.006.

67 "Stillbirth." Cleveland Clinic, n.d., my.clevelandclinic.org/health/diseases/9685-stillbirth.

due to delivery. And if a C-section occurred, pain itching, and discomfort in the surgery site may arise.

Connect Deeper. The grieving process for a stillbirth is one which is unique in every way. When someone experiences a stillbirth, there is no one who can more intimately touch the experience of loss than the one who knew this being the most intimately, the mother/parent.

To honor this loss, create a simple ceremony by gathering one or two items which represent the baby and the time you had together. Place them on your altar while saying their name aloud. Write down or say things you wish to share with their spirit that you have not said aloud or yet written. Do this in your own time. Ask your partner or a friend to participate in this ceremony if it feels most supportive.

Part Two: Womb Herbalism 101

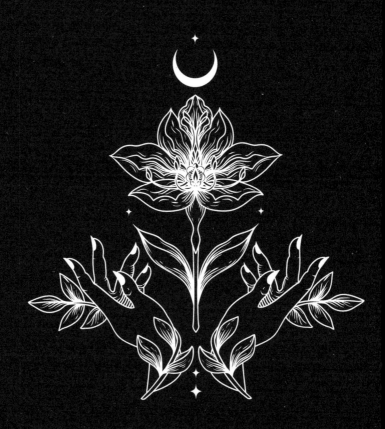

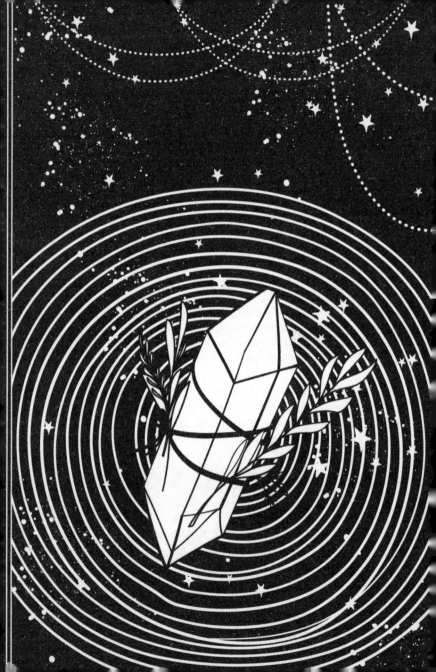

Introduction: Herbalism, the Folk Method, and Honoring the Wisdom

*T*he wild ways in which we work with our wombspace is a space heavily saturated in herbalism. Herbalism is the study and use of wild, medicinal plants. Whether you've realized it or not, you've practiced herbalism. Peppermint tea is herbalism. Oregano added to a dish is herbalism. Using rose water on your face is herbalism. And throughout these pages, I will unveil to you how learning and practicing herbalism can deeply nourish and support the womb system.

Whether you have an apothecary or have never made tea with anything other than a bag, the pages to come will prepare you to start using the plants reviewed in this book in intentional, medicinal ways.

Many of the herbs discussed are gentle, but effective. Some herbs are more strong, and require active monitoring of the body's response to their use. While I make a point of providing you with information that differentiates between when an herb is gentle or more strong, body literacy and awareness is key. When trying any new herb or supplement, I highly recommend doing a body scan from head to toe, noting patterns in tissue states, tension/tightness, and overall feeling in each part of your body. Be aware of how you feel before and after you use a new herb. I will repeat this sentiment often throughout the course of these pages, as it is important: Before using an herb, be sure to check for any contraindications with prescription drugs you may be taking and consult a healthcare provider.

I most often use and teach the folk tradition of herbalism, called folk herbalism. This is the tradition I will be drawing from in this book. Folk herbalism is the most user-friendly and age-old method of herbalism, for it is the tradition of using plants in a way that is community-oriented, based on cultural traditions. It's the method our ancestors used when they made their seasonal herbal tonics, as was the common way until recently. As the folk method is so accessible, typically using "parts" as measurements, it is easy to make herbal medicines and extractions with items you likely have on hand. For example, if you venture into a field with a jar and apple cider vinegar, you could come back with violet flower–infused vinegars. I like the freedom and simplicity of this. And that's why it's the method I prefer using.

Some other types of herbalism include clinical and community herbalism, which require deeper study and practice, often with the inclusion of formal trainings and apprenticeships. See the appendix for herb schools and programs which I have either personally attended or think highly of in regards to the material offered.

Chapter Five: Herbal Energetics

*I*f you've ever googled, "What herbs will heal [fill in health issue]," only to use said herb and have it not work for your body? There are many reasons as to why this might happen, but it may largely be due to a mismatch of herbal energetics. Within this field of study, each herb, tissue state, and our individual bodies have their own unique energy, which all lie on a spectrum. Understanding this spectrum is important to understanding the ways in which one herb may be properly applied. It also sheds light on why all herbs are not for all people.

This part of herbalism is nuanced and takes much study and practice to deeply understand. To properly use herbs that will effectively work with your body, this is a topic that must be understood at an introductory level. And that's what this section is: an introduction to herbal energetics. As I've insinuated, there is much more to learn about this subject, but I believe you will be able to appropriately proceed with using herbs at a baseline level after assessing and implementing this knowledge.

When applying herbs to our bodies, we are trying to achieve or maintain balance, holding the homeostasis needle steady or causing it to tip in other directions. Because of this ability, even the most gentle herbs are potent and hold the ability to direct your body into a different state that may or may not be supportive when used over a period of time.

The energetics categories we denote for our constitution, our tissue states, and the herbs we use includes: Warming/Cooling, Drying/Damp, and Tense/Lax. Notice that each category includes a pair of opposites. However, it's important to remember that the herbal energetics for each plant remain on a spectrum whose expression may be brought forward more depending on your personal energetics and/or the way you use them. In some cases, herbs may be applied to nourish opposing body constitutions/tissues to bring balance.

Before beginning with herbs, it is important to know your constitution and energetic state of your tissues. Your constitution is the normal, everyday state of your body. If you're familiar with Ayurveda medicine, you may have heard of the three doshas, which are body type constitutions: Vata, Pitta, or Kapha. Alternatively, you may have heard of the body types described in western medicine: Endomorph, Ectomorph, and Mesomorph. The following pages will help you understand what type of constitution/tissue state you have.[68]

In addition to knowing your constitution, you must consider and note the tissue state of the areas that are imbalanced. While keeping in mind that it's imperative to consider the root causes of health issues when applying herbs, we do want to choose herbs which will directly support bringing health to the area of concentration. Typically, tissue states will be prone towards your constitution. There are exceptions to this viewpoint when something acute occurs, such as a burn, a poison ivy rash, diarrhea, or scrapes/cuts.

For example: You are a person who has a warm, moist, and lax constitution that also experiences seasonal allergies. It may be likely that the allergy symptoms appear as feeling excessively hot and congested with loose tissue states in your upper respiratory tract.

In this case, we may want to apply drying, cooling herbs such as Nettle and Goldenrod. If you would apply herbs that promote moistening or warming properties, this could push the

---

68 If you are unsure and would like a supportive resource in finding if you have chosen the right ways to describe your body type, consider taking the dosha quiz from Banyan Botanicals: banyanbotanicals.com/info/dosha-quiz/. This resource will assist you in finding your "resting" constitution and is full of insight to enlighten you on a variety of ways you can work with your body in a holistic sense.

tissue states or your overall constitution into a place where the herbs will do more harm than good.

As you can see, herbal energetics are important to consider for efficacy! So, let's dive in.

Below, each constitution and tissue state is listed alongside common factors associated with it. I've also included a small list of plants that may nourish and support that specific constitution/tissue state as well as herbs that are associated with its specific energy.

If you need more support in understanding these concepts, I highly recommend extending your studies in herbalism with one of the resources located in the appendix.

Warm

At the most extreme, a warm constitution/tissue state denotes qualities of hyperactivity. Essentially, this stage tends towards overexertion of body function. At its subtle state, it looks like a general excitement and steady energy and may include some of the qualities listed below.

A warm constitution/tissue state may look like:
- A fast metabolism
- A red face
- Excessive inflammation
- Anxiety
- Jitters
- Temper
- Overheating
- Allergic reactions that are fiery, red, swollen
- Excessive sweating
- Strong appetite
- Feeling hot at night when sleeping
- Easily aggravated/emotional/intense
- Anger

- A hyperactive immune system
- Stabbing pain
- Insomnia
- Sprains

Herbs that may cool down and balance a warm state include: Linden, Milky Oats, Mint, Hibiscus, Rose, and Chickweed.

Application Example: It is a hot day. You are a person with an already warm constitution. You are excessively sweating, aggravated, and overheating. You may choose to drink any of the herbs listed above and feel the relief of your body cooling down.

Warming herbs are typically stimulating, are circulatory-focused, assist in movement (especially for resisting stagnation), and may bring relief to cold states/conditions.

Herbs that are considered WARM (to a varying degree) include: Cayenne, Horseradish, Turmeric, Ginger Root, Garlic, Cinnamon, Garlic, Black Pepper, Elecampane Root.

Cold

Cold constitutions and tissue states are usually seen and experienced as qualities of depression. They are underactive and prone towards deficiency.

A cold constitution/tissue state may look like:

- A pale complexion
- Slow digestion/movement
- Tending towards depression, sadness, being withdrawn, and quiet states
- Extremities that are frequently cold or finding it hard to keep heat in the body
- Not sweating easily
- Low appetite
- Low immune system function
- Brain fog
- Being less likely to have strong reactions

- Dull, slow aching pain
- Bruising

Herbs that may bring balance to a cold constitution/tissue state are going to be warming, spicy, aromatic, and stimulating. This includes: Thyme, Bee Balm, Ginger Root, Cardamom, Turmeric, Black Pepper.

Application Example: You are experiencing intense menstrual cramps with blood clots. This communication from your body signals that you may be having difficulty with stagnancy in your uterus, which is energetically cold. You consider using ginger root tea, because it is warming, stimulating, and known to assist in moving stagnation in menses.

Herbs that are considered cold tend towards cooling, relieving high fevers/overheated bodies, may be sedative in nature, and are likely to slow down the energy and flow.

Herbs that are considered COLD (to a varying degree) include: Violet, Linden, Dandelion Root, Chickweed, Burdock Root, Peppermint, Self-Heal, and Echinacea.

Damp

Damp constitution/tissue states can be experienced as places where excessive fluids and stagnation are present.

A damp constitution/tissue state may look like:
- Sweating easily
- Being prone to mucus
- More water retention in the body
- Varicose veins
- Hemorrhoids
- Edema
- Stagnation in circulation
- Swelling in joints
- Bloating
- Diarrhea

- A heavy feeling in body and emotionally

Herbs that may bring balance to a damp constitution/tissue state are either going to be drying to the entire body (if taken internally), which is going to directly affect a person's body type/constitution or they will be specific to the tissue state via toning actions due to astringency.

Herbs that may assist in damp constitutions include: Nettle, Goldenrod, and Chamomile, Black Tea.

Herbs that may assist in damp tissue states include: Yarrow, Witch Hazel, Sage, and Rose.

Application Example: Rose Hydrosol may be used as a toner in skincare, on sunburns, and to assist the healing process with weeping wounds. When edema is present, Nettle Leaf may be of assistance, as is it wholly drying to the constitution.

Herbs that are considered damp are soothing to dried, irritated tissues and are often described as mucilaginous and demulcent.

Herbs that are considered DAMP (to a varying degree) include: Marshmallow Root, Aloe Vera, Linden Leaf, Violet, Chickweed, and Slippery Elm.

Dry

Dry constitution/tissue states can be experienced as places where hardening, separation, atrophy, and loss of strength are present. Fluids are not being properly retained, or not properly stocked, in the body.

A dry constitution/tissue state may look like:
- Dry skin/hair
- Brittle nails
- Constipation
- Nervous tension
- Feeling frazzled

- Chapped lips
- Stiff joints

Herbs that may bring balance to a dry constitution/tissue state are either going to be moistening, demulcent, lubricating, or mucilaginous. Sometimes introducing herbs that cause secretion of more fluids from the tissues can further exacerbate a dry condition. We want the body to keep the fluids in the tissues for deep nourishment.

Adaptogens such as Ashwagandha, Licorice, and Milky Oats will assist in overall stimulation of moistening qualities to the body as a whole. Demulcents, such as Marshmallow Root, Aloe, Chickweed, Plantain, Violet, and Slippery Elm, provide assistance to tissue states that need their mucilaginous qualities as soon as possible.

Application Example: A dry, scratchy throat may greatly enjoy a cold infusion[69] of Marshmallow root as its extremely moistening qualities can be soothing to dry, irritated conditions. A person who has experienced chronic dry qualities, such as a frazzled, nervous tension mental state, may greatly benefit from Milky Oats infusions.

Herbs that are considered dry are soothing to draining to excess fluids, and may tighten and tone the constitution/tissue state.

Herbs that are considered DRY (to a varying degree) include: Dandelion Leaf, Cayenne, Nettle Leaf, Raspberry Leaf, Cleavers, and Lavender.

Tense

Tense constitution/tissue states can be experienced as places where extreme tightness and restriction will cause tissues to degrade, not receive proper circulation, and become more rigid. It impedes the flow of energy, fluids, and overall circulation.

A tense constitution/tissue state may look like:

---

69 Read more about what an herbal infusion is in Chapter 7.

- Stiff muscles
- Irritability
- Constipation
- Muscle spasms
- Tremors and chills
- Issues with elimination
- Stiff joints
- Chronic cramping
- Scar tissue
- Lack of flexibility in joints and muscles
- Tension headaches

Herbs that may bring balance to a damp constitution/tissue state are either going to be relaxing, antispasmodic, sedative, or dispersive. Herbs that have these qualities include Kava Kava, Passionflower, Poppy, Peach, Cannabis, and Chamomile.

Application Example: A person is experiencing issues with properly digesting the food they're eating. They are constantly irritable and constipated. They may take Chamomile, which is both relaxing and great in assisting with digestion.

Herbs that are tense in energetics are usually astringent, tonifying, and tightening to tissues. Herbs that are categorized as assisting in TENSE effects include: Horse Chestnut, Witch Hazel, Rose, Oak Bark.

Lax

Lax constitution/tissue states can be experienced as places where there is lack of form, tightness, and tone. In its easiest sense lax = overly relaxed. Elasticity may be lost, skin may be flabby and shapeless, and an over-abundance of fluid loss may be present.

A lax constitution/tissue state may look like:
- Organ prolapse
- Excessive diarrhea, vomiting, bleeding, and sweating

- Loose tissue
- Being prone to over-worrying/anxiety
- Being bad with setting boundaries
- Hemorrhoids

Herbs that may bring balance to a lax constitution/tissue state are either going to assist the body in tightening, toning, or bringing strength back to the tissues where there is too much laxness.

Herbs that may assist in lax tissue states include: Black Tea, Witch Hazel, Nettle Leaf, Raspberry Leaf, Oak, and Rose.

Application Example: A person is experiencing a bothersome hemorrhoid. They may find relief by making a sitz bath with a cooled down tea of raspberry leaf and rose petals.

Herbs that are considered LAX encourage dispersion of tension and constriction and are usually anti-spasmodic. This includes: Valerian, Cannabis, Wood Betony, and Lemon Balm.

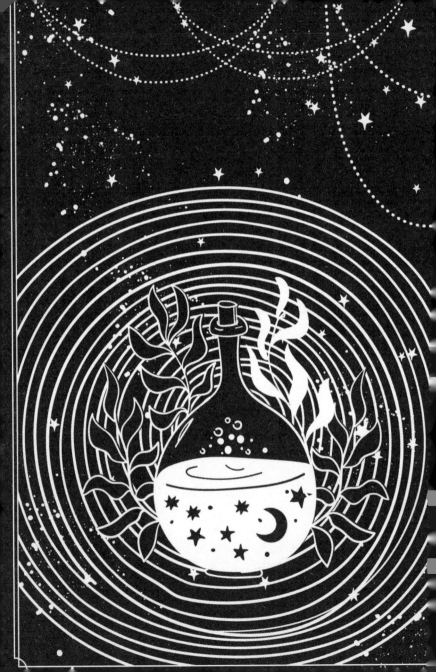

Chapter Six: Safety First—Herbalism Best Practices for Every Womb

Safety and Herbs

*H*erbs are safe to use. But not all herbs are safe to use for all people, conditions, lengths of time, or prescription pills. I do my best at noting contraindications. However, not all supplements, herbalists, or social media posts do this. I insist that you go the extra mile in doing your due diligence when it comes to research if you have a health condition or take prescription medications that may experience an interaction with herbs. I highly recommend utilizing the *Herbal Materia Medica* manual by Michael Moore, who was a western herbalist. This incredible resource can be found for free on his website and offers information on the safety and dosage recommendations for over 500 major botanical medicines (swsbm.com/ManualsMM/MatMed5.pdf). In addition, as always, talk to your health care provider before starting any new usage of herbs or supplements.

If you are unsure if an herb is right for you: Don't take it.

If you experience a headache, nausea, diarrhea, vomiting, rashes, or hives from an herb that you have taken—do NOT proceed. Call the poison control center immediately.

This is not to scare, but to inform you. I have been using a wide variety of herbs for well over a decade and have not experienced any volatile reactions to what I or my clients have taken. But, we are all different. I recommend that you are certain you have herbs from a trusted source, that you do your research on any contraindications, and start slowly in using any herbs.

Dosing and Herbs

Dosing herbs properly, safely, and effectively is an art. One that you can learn to do as long as you listen to your body. I suggest that you start with small doses, especially if you have not used an herb before. This means, a small sip from a cup of tea before drinking it in its entirety. If using a tincture,[70] try a few drops in your mouth, close your eyes and focus on any immediate shifts you may notice. Be certain that your body doesn't have any intense reactions after imbibing the herb before proceeding to a higher dose.

When using a tonic plant, which is one that can be used over a period of time to rebuild or maintain health, a standard dose for a tincture is 2 to 3 droppers[71] full in water/soda/liquid 2 to 3 times a day at its highest dose. For a tonic tea, you may drink one cup 2 to 3 times a day. You may still reap the benefits of the herb if you decide to take a smaller dose, such as 2 to 3 droppers full of a tincture one time a day, or 1 cup of tea one time a day as long as there is consistency in this usage. Listen to your body's cues and adjust as needed.

Herbs which are used in acute situations—such as colds/flus, constipation (unless chronic), food poisoning, or first aid instances—may call for a stronger type of herb. With this, the dosages above may be used, but for shorter periods of time: days or two weeks at a time, instead of daily for months.

Overall, whenever dosing herbs, please remember the protocols in the Safety and Herbs section. Not all herbs are meant to be taken as a tonic. Not all herbs should be taken, or may be tolerated, by all people. Some plants should be used

---

70 A tincture is an extract made from plant material in a solvent, typically alcohol. We review tinctures in Chapter 7.

71 In folk herbalism, you will often see "a dropper full" as a recommended dosage. This refers to the tincture bottle dropper, which may vary in dosage depending on the tincture bottle size when squeezed. Typically, 45-60 droplets can be seen as an adjacent equivalent to "a dropper full."

for two weeks with a large break, which could span multiple months. Or, two weeks and then taking a break for a month and then continuing after the break. Or, some should be used for a few days at a time only in acute situations. As you can see, dosing herbs that are not tonic can become complicated. This is a great example as to why googling herbs to address symptoms oftentimes produces poor results.

If you are unsure of how to tell if an herb is gentle enough for prolonged use or a strong herb that should be used with more caution, I highly recommend doing further research on the herb you are choosing to use by obtaining a book that includes details specifically on herbs, their dosages, and historical use. Suggestions for these types of books can be found in the appendix. Additionally, I highly recommend consulting and working with a clinical herbalist[72] when working on complex herbal protocols, as they will be able to offer more refined recommendations on dosing and formulation.

Examples of herbs typically used as tonics largely include nourishing herbs. We discuss this class of herbs in the section on herbal infusions, which can be found in Chapter 7. A few examples of herbs which should be used with caution—for only a specific time period and dosage and with mindfulness—include ephedra, lobelia, sena, pokeweed, comfrey, wormwood, kava kava, and licorice root.

Sourcing and Herbs

You've found an herb you're interested in. It feels aligned energetically. You have no health conditions or medications that would negatively interact with the plant. It feels supportive to your system and holistically sound. But, you want the herb to work. And that's where quality comes into play, which is

---

72 Locate a clinical herbalist near you through a local apothecary, wellness store, or through the Registered Herbalist (RH) database on americanherbalistsguild.com.

incredibly important when it comes to herbalism. You want your herbs to smell, look, and feel like they were preserved with care.

We don't all have access to wild harvesting our own plants or growing our own. However, with the popularity of herbalism, access to herbs—even freshly grown herbs— has become more prevalent. Below are some options for finding herbs to use.

Locavore[73]
Local, local, local—always choose this option if it is possible and accessible.

You can source herbs locally in several different ways. Go to a local apothecary. Buy bulk herbs from herb farms in your bioregion. Check your farmers markets for herb farmers that sell freshly cut plants.

Bulk Herbs from Small Farmers
If you are not able to locate a local herb farmer, or if they do not have the herbs you wish to source, consider purchasing herbs from a small herb farm. The quality of small farms is, many times, superior to some of the bigger names. As always, do your research on the sourcing and growing practices of the farm you are considering. Find out who is growing the plants and how. Are they using sustainable, regenerative practices? Are they organic? How old are the herbs? You don't want to buy bulk herbs harvested in 2015 that have been sprayed with pesticides, as their medicine will not offer much for you or the person you are offering it to.

It's also important to know that if a plant is available, it doesn't always mean it is being ethically sold. It is still your responsibility to check the status of the plant to ensure you are not buying something that shouldn't be offered for commerce in the first place. If you find the store/farmers are selling at-risk

---

73 A locavore is someone who eats and uses foods and medicinal plants that are grown within their direct bioregion, typically within 100 miles of where they live.

plants, ask questions and do research. Find out if the practices they're using will ensure the sustainability of the plant. As witches, it's our responsibility to do this research, as this not only looks out for the health of our planet, but is in the vein of being spiritually attuned to the gravity of failing to do so, which ultimately results in the imbalance of the ecosystem.

Bigger Retailers

Many apothecaries, co-ops, and big name websites will carry bulk herbs from bigger retailers such as Mountain Rose Herbs, Starwest Botanicals, and Frontier Herbs. If these brands are who you choose to source your herbs through, you can rest easy knowing that they are known for offering organic herbs that are safe to use.

Foraging: Ethically and Responsibly Harvesting Wild Plants

Making your own herbal medicines is a magick I wish all could experience. These medicines instantly connect us with the natural world, our bioregions, and the plants who support and nourish the Earth we call home. Profound healing takes place when using oils and teas and salves you have used your own hands to harvest and craft.

If making your own herbal medicines, chances are you are harvesting your plants in the wild or through a farm that offers fresh harvests or you-pick options. Or, you may have dry plant material that you wish to create infused oils, tinctures, or teas with. Before making herbal medicine with plants or mushrooms you've gathered, there are things to know when it comes to harvesting wild medicines and sourcing cultivated herbs in responsible, ethical ways.

Our aim in foraging is not just to take from the lands, but to find ways we can sustainably support the ecosystems we visit and live in. With this in mind, below is a quick rundown of what I consider to be the most important things to know for a responsible harvest of edible and medicinal plants.

Build a Reciprocal Relationship with the Land

Before embarking on a plant harvest, consider what type of relationship you have with the land you will be harvesting from. If you aren't able to forage in an area you live in or are frequently near, make time to regularly visit the land you seek to forage from. This is the first step in establishing a relationship. Like any relationship in life, it takes time, patience, and awareness. Building this relationship is not only an ethical and safe thing to do, but it is an important spiritual aspect of gathering plants in general, one that shows pure intention. Do not underestimate the power of this. There is magick in taking the time to learn and choose what is most respectful to the land, rather than prioritizing speed and only focusing on what we want from the land. This process is not only the ethical thing to do but it is also something we do for ourselves and our place in the web of life—for we are all connected.

Put another way, if we do not know the lands we are harvesting from, how are we to know they are safe, clean places to forage from? How will we know if the lands we have chosen are places that are already being threatened by overharvesting? How can we ensure we are making the highest quality medicines by making sure our processes and practices are intentional?

In crafting wild medicines, our aim is to engage in reciprocity. We are looking for ways to both gather from the land and give back with reverence to all it offers us. We can lean into this reciprocity with the land by participating in the rest of the practices in this list.

Know the Status of the Plant

It is incredibly important to check the status of the plant you wish to harvest in the wild. Simply seeing an abundant stand of a plant in the wild doesn't mean it is abundant elsewhere. Some questions to ask here:

Is the plant at risk or endangered? Should you be looking for ways to re-establish it in the wild vs. harvesting it? How long does this plant take to grow into maturity?

United Plant Savers offers information on plants that are critically endangered, at risk, or in review of being at risk and is a great resource to learn more information on these plants, as well as ways to re-populate the ones specific to your bioregion. Familiarize yourself with the plants which are endangered or at risk so that you can work to not harvest or buy products with these plants in them.

Examples of plants that have been over-harvested and require TIME to grow healthy stands: White Sage, Ginseng, Osha, Solomon's Seal.

If you are buying from a bulk retailer or farm that is selling at risk plants, do research on their practices. Ensure the plant was farmed and not wild harvested.

Ultimately, it would be best for us to find out what invasive species are thriving in our area. Harvest these plants. Invasive species compete with local plants and are typically incredibly abundant. EatTheInvaders.org is a wonderful resource which may help you locate the ones active in your bioregion. There is Garlic Mustard in the spring. Rosa multiflora in the midwest summers. And, oodles of blackberry on the west coast. Plants which all carry rich medicinal and edible value.

Harvest Mindfully

Harvest the correct part of the plant for the season you are in. A plant may offer a different kind of medicine depending on the month and season that you harvest it. For example, tree bark should be harvested, with some exceptions, during early spring or fall when the energetic vitality of a tree is at its peak. Also, some plants contain medicine in one part and are poisonous in their other parts. Avoid harvesting plants in the morning when dew is present or if they have been rained on as the added water will make it difficult to adequately dry the material, or may spoil herbal medicine.

Example A: Elder leaves, bark, and seeds of the fruit contain cyanogenic glycosides, which are known to be poisonous and will likely induce vomiting. However, their flowers and ripe berries have been used in herbal medicines for centuries and are harvested in the spring (flowers) and summer (berries).

Example B: Dandelion leaves are harvested in the early spring when they are fresh and more tender. While they can be harvested in the summer months, they may be tough and require cooking. Dandelion root may be harvested from the fall months to spring. I find their bitter qualities shine in the autumnal months after a few frosts. However, dandelions' spring roots are rich in inulin and may be used as a more palatable food.

Be Mindful of the Amount You Are Harvesting

A general rule in harvesting wild edible and medicinal plants is to only take one-tenth of what you see. Intentionally spread out your harvesting locations and be sure to not take too much from any single area. Aim to leave the area as if you were never there. Although cut stalks and missing flowers will be left behind, be mindful that your harvesting is carefully dispersed.

Over-harvesting will leave ecosystems and plant stands devastated and threatened. These plants exist not only for our personal use, but for the animals, insects, and other plants who thrive off their existence. To respect plant life and all of life is to leave it in a healthy state.

Put Intention in the Act of Harvesting

This may look like asking the plant for permission before you harvest it. Close your eyes. Breathe in and out until you find a place of quiet inside. Hover your hands over the plant/tree/ mushroom or gently place your hands on it. Ask aloud (or mentally through your hands) if you have permission to harvest from this stand or tree. Listen for the no or a yes. Plants are living beings who, despite not having nervous systems or brains, have consciousness and visceral life force and as such, should be offered respect during and after the harvest.[74]

If you don't know how to tell if a plant is saying "Yes, harvest me" or "No," I suggest visiting that plant multiple times before actually taking any part of the plant. Get to know the area it surrounds. Is it the only plant stand of its kind? What animals and insects surround this place and plant? Does the land where you stand feel at peace? Deep awareness and inner quietude is asked for to find the answers to these questions.

From the center of your being, where we find our gut answers, a feeling will arise, offering you your yes or no.[75] If all you sense in the experience of plant harvesting are abundant yes's, I invite you to tune in and listen more deeply. This type of deep listening takes practice to hone. Intention is the most important thing here. Use discernment. Gather lightly or not at all if you are unsure if you should be harvesting from a particular plant stand or tree.

When you do harvest, I urge you to adopt the practice of leaving an offering of tobacco, water, prayer, or song to the area. This energy is then infused into the space as a gift that

---

74 "Awareness and Integrated Information Theory Identify Plant Meristems as Sites of Conscious Activity," *Springer*, 2021, link.springer.com/article/10.1007/ s00709-021-01633-1.
75 Working with plants in such an intentional way demands that we tune into deep layers of ourselves. This work will not only be felt in the plant medicines that you craft, but it will echo into other parts of your life, offering deeper intuitive knowing and wisdom.

recognizes to take with deep awareness is to respect and honor the place that offers its medicines.

Seed Scattering

Seed scattering, when appropriate, is a way to ensure a plant remains active and alive in an area.

If you have confirmed that the plant whose seeds you wish to scatter is NOT an invasive plant, but a local plant who encourages the bioregion to remain diverse, scatter their seeds. It's important to always do your research prior to taking seeds and scattering them to ensure you are doing no harm.

From this, consider propagating starts of the plant and repopulating them in an area where construction, damage, or over-harvesting has taken place. There are many native plants that are in need of more people to do this responsibly.

Safety of harvesting in the Wild

When I first started harvesting wild plants, my family thought I had officially lost it. My dad was convinced I was collecting a death salad every time I left the house with a basket and some shearers. And, considering his plant knowledge of the woods behind our house, I can't blame him. Luckily, I had an excellent mentor who showed me the way to plant identification and the safety of harvesting in the wild, or even from your garden. If there is anything you pay attention to when it comes to harvesting plants, let it be in this section. (Although, of course, I would be remiss to not say I think every section is absolutely important.) For safety, there are a few rules that should absolutely be followed and considered before embarking on a harvest.

Familiarize Yourself with the Poisonous Plants Lookalikes

Sometimes a plant that has a poisonous lookalike will grow near or next to each other. Or, they may not grow next to each other at all. It is important to be able to positively ID any plant that you harvest. Knowing which plants could be confused with the plant you are harvesting is paramount to safe harvesting practices.

An example: Wild Carrot, which is also known as Queen Anne's Lace, and Poison Hemlock may look very similar to someone who does not know these plants individually. Hemlock is poisonous and can be lethal if ingested, while Queen Anne's Lace has multiple medicinal uses.

Acquire a Guidebook and Watch Plant ID Videos
These are invaluable resources that will tell you what a plant looks like, what types of environments it grows in, as well as what parts of the plant are in season for harvesting. They will also usually make note of what parts of the plant aren't edible or, if the plant has a lookalike.

Consider Where You Are Harvesting From
Harvesting from a safe, clean area far from toxic waste plants, polluted lands or waterways, roadsides, and areas that are sprayed with pesticides is an important factor to consider. We are making medicine with these plants, and many of them will soak up or be infused with the pollution in the areas where they grow.

Putting It All Together: Questions to Ask Before Foraging/Harvesting
The safety of your harvest doesn't involve only considering the safety of yourself and anyone else who may consume your medicine, but the safety of the plants too.

To help you figure out if you are charging forth with a harvest that is both safe and ethically done, answer this checklist of questions before you get started.

Questions to consider before harvesting plants in the wild...
- What herb are you looking for?
- What is its Latin name? This is important to avoid confusion when someone is showing you a plant. (Example: Some people call clover chickweed, when it is NOT chickweed nor should be used like chickweed in many circumstances.)
- Is it endangered/at risk?
- What does it look like? Be specific. Very specific. Take notes. If you're unsure, don't harvest it.
- Where does it grow?
- Does it have any poisonous lookalikes?
- What part of the plant are you looking to harvest?
- Are you harvesting the plant part in the correct season?
- What do you plan on doing with the plant?
- How soon will you be able to process[76] the plant?
- Is the plant healthy? Have bugs eaten the leaves and/or infested other parts of the plant?
- Does the plant look vibrant and at the peak of its prime?
- Do you have the correct tools to harvest this plant?

Once you've answered these questions with full confidence... you're ready!

Processing Your Herbs

Once you've harvested herbs, you will want to process them as soon as possible. The longer plants aren't stored properly, the quicker they degrade.

For processing plants whose leaves, flowers, seeds, or roots you wish to keep for storage or medicine, there are a few ways to go about this. First, consider these questions: What will you be using these plants for? Are you drying them for later use? Or, will you be making medicine with them fresh? This determines how you will proceed with processing.

---

76 We will review how to process plants in the next section.

Something that will be repeated often in these pages: Water will create conditions for mold, degradation, and rancidity. Do not wash leaves, flowers, seeds, bark, and berries after harvesting. With this in mind, avoid harvesting plants that are excessively dirty and muddy, with the exception of roots. Roots are the only plant material that are washed before using in herbal medicine or storage. To make medicine right away, start by sorting through your plants. For every harvest, no matter how you plan on using them, it is absolutely necessary to go through EVERY individual plant/leaf/flower/seed/root that you have harvested. Discard any plant material that isn't in prime shape and any other plants you may find intertwined with the one you intended to harvest. Keep an eye out for bugs, fungus, and mold. Do not keep any plant material that contains these things—it will not give you the medicine you seek and it will degrade any good material you did harvest.

Take extra care to be thorough in this step. This will ensure the safety and potency of the medicine you are creating. A different species of plant (or bugs) will almost always end up intertwined in the plants you have gathered, as we are extracting the wild from the wild. Set the bugs free and return plant material back to the earth. Or, consider processing your plants in the area where you harvest them, as this will yield the best results for all.

To process roots: Start by soaking the roots in a bowl or 5-gallon jug of water. As the dirt loosens up, scrub them clean. Wash and scrub with clean water multiple times until the water runs clear. Chop roots into small chunks or shavings. This is optimal for both drying and to make medicine with, as it exposes more surface of the root.

To process bark: Using a sharp knife with strokes that flow away from your body, strip the top layer of the bark, leaves, and any debris from the branch. Continue to strip the bark of its soft, thick, and moist bark, which will contain the medicinal compounds. Small twigs may be used as well, but will create a weaker medicinal extraction.

Drying Your Herbs

Drying your herbs with care allows you to maintain their aromatic and medicinal qualities, which potentially can last for years. This means more robust medicines and deeply delicious teas.

The MOST important thing to remember when drying herbs is that moisture is the enemy. We want to ensure that every bit of the plant material is completely dried before they are placed in storage. As mentioned above, if moisture is present, mold and degradation will follow.

The following drying options may be applied to flowers, leaves, berries, bark, and roots.

Dehydrate

Dehydrating your harvest will provide you with a more swift drying time as well as a higher standard of preserved herbs. The quicker a plant dries, the higher quality it will remain. Dehydration is the go-to method if drying herbs that are delicate or contain aromatic qualities you wish to more deeply preserve.

Using a dehydrator, lay a thin layer of leaves/flowers/berries/bark/roots on dehydrator trays. Dehydrate according to the specific dehydrator's instructions for herbs. For most leaves and flowers, dehydrate between 95°F and 115°F for 4 to 6 hours. For seeds, bark, or roots, dehydrate between 110°F and 125°F. Temperatures may need to be adjusted depending on humidity of the environment you are in. After that time has elapsed, check the plant material for moisture. Continue to dehydrate as needed. This will vary from plant to plant.

If you do not have a dehydrator, and this is a method you wish to explore, you may be able to effectively use your convection oven. Technically, this will bake the herbs, but will ultimately result in drying them out. Set the oven temperature for 170° F, or its lowest setting, for leaves and flowers and 200°F for bark, roots, seeds, and berries. After one hour, check the plant material to find the rate at which they are drying. Flip the plant material if needed. Continue to bake until completely dry. The plant material must be cooled before storing them in airtight jars or bags.

Drying Rack/Trays
If space permits, consider getting a drying rack or hanging trays/baskets. You will simply lay your plant material in a thin layer on the rack/trays in a well-ventilated space. Depending on your environment, it may take days or weeks for your plants to fully dry. Check moisture levels often and consider using a dehumidifier to support the process.

Tie the Stalks Together and Hang Them
For this method, you will need twine/string and a place to hang your herbs, preferably near a window or well-ventilated area. Place 3 to 4 stalks of the plant together in a bunch, tying them together at the base of where you cut. Be sure to not overcrowd the plants as you will want them to have space to dry. This will vary plant to plant.

Hang them from a line or space, placing the bottom of the stalks to the sky, leaving the rest of the plant matter dangling towards the Earth.

Drying time can range from a few days to a week or two, depending on the humidity in your home/environment and the density of the plant. Check their moisture level often. When stems start to snap, this is a good indicator that the plant material is dry. This method is ideal for flowers and leaves.

The Paper Bag Method

If you do not have excessive space or time, this method will come in handy. It's worth noting that this method will degrade your plant material more than the others. But, it works if you are in a pinch. All you need are paper bags, patience, and a commitment to being active in the drying process. This method calls for herbs that are already processed as full stalks will not allow for thorough drying in bags.

Divide your harvest into paper bags, being sure to not overcrowd. Fill the bags no more than one-fourth of the way full. To start, leave the tops of the bags open, tossing the plant material around with your hands, lightly, at least 2 to 3 times a day. When I dry plants in this method, I place the bags in the common area and shake the bags every time I walk past.

After a few days of drying, you may want to close the bags. Continue to toss the plant matter around throughout the day, while opening the bags to check moisture levels at least once a day.

Storing Your Herbs

You've harvested your herbs. You've processed them. They are now dry. It's time to store them well so that your hard work and their medicine may be preserved.

Label

Write a detailed label. Always. Especially when making medicines or storing herbs. A good, precise label will prevent guesswork and keep things organized. With this, you will never have to figure out what you've made or placed in a random jar, because you'll have a label that does that for you. For every medicine you make and every plant you dry and store, include a label with this information:

- common plant name

- Latin name
- the date
- the location you made your medicine in or harvested the plant from
- life/lunar details (As in, what phase of the moon did you make your medicine in? Was there an eclipse? A new moon? A holiday? Maybe there was a thunderstorm...or a heartache...or a celebration. Or a detailed reason for why you made the medicine.)

Example:

Lilac Honey

Syringa vulgaris

06/24/2021

Cleveland, Ohio

Full Moon, Strawberry!

Where and How to Store Your Herbs?

Glass Jars vs. Paper Bags

I consider glass to be the best option for storing herbs long-term: mason jars, airtight jars, repurposed food jars. Glass will protect from moisture/critters and degradation of the plant matter.

Paper bags act as suitable storage in the short-term. With prolonged use, they lead to excessive dryness of the herbs, which will cause them to break down and lose medicinal quality. If this is your only option, be sure to store the bags in a cool, dark space.

Location

Sunlight and heat degrade herbs, whether they are stored in glass, plastic, or paper. Place herbs and extractions in a dark, cool closet. Or a shelf that is shielded from direct sunlight.

Your Equipment

The folk tradition of making plant medicines is grand in part because of its simplicity. You won't need many things to start. However, it is important to prioritize the quality of the vessels and tools you will be using.

Containers

Water preparations[77] and oil infusions are best made in glass, stainless steel, clay, or enamel vessels. It is best to avoid plastic and "no stick" pots and pans when possible, especially when doing something such as medicine making, which is an extractive process. For other medicinal preparations, such as tinctures, oxymels, or infused honeys, I find it wise and best to stick to glass.

Menstruum

The menstruum is the vehicle for your plant medicine. Meaning, in herbal honeys, honey is the menstruum. In vinegar infusions, vinegar is the menstruum.

We want our menstruum to be of the highest quality possible. Organic, raw honey. Organic apple cider vinegar. Oil that is organic, cold-pressed, and unrefined. Alcohol which is organic and potentially gluten free, if necessary.

Wax/Parchment Paper

As you make herbal medicines, you will need wax or parchment paper to act as a barrier between the lids and your medicine.[78] Menstruums such as vinegar and alcohol corrode metal lids over time and will leech into the extractions. Placing a piece of

---

77 Water preparations include teas, tisanes, infusions, and decoctions, which we will go over in Chapter 7.

78 To practice this, place one small square of wax or parchment paper on top of the mouth of the jar. Next, you will fit the lid on top. You may need to readjust to make it fit in a snug and secure way. Turn jar upside down to test its tightness and ensure no liquids escape.

wax/parchment paper at the mouth of your jars is an important step in preventing this from happening.

Labels

If you aim for aesthetically pleasing jars, you may want to purchase sticker labels and markers. Or, you can simply write on a piece of paper and tape it to the jars you use.

Other Tools

Other tools it would be wise to keep on hand include:

- wooden chopsticks (for stirring medicines/poking out air bubbles in honey and oil extractions)
- a scale (in case you wish to create more accurate medicines where you take note of how much plant material/menstruum you are using)
- a knife/cutting board (for chopping up plant material such as roots or for peeling off bark from branches)
- cheesecloth (for straining plant material when they are done infusing)
- pop top bottles, amber bottles, and metal tins for salve
- glass jars and metal tins to pour your infused medicines inside of
- a variety of funnels for pouring liquids into jars and tincture bottles

Part Three: Herbalism & Holistic Therapies for Every Womb

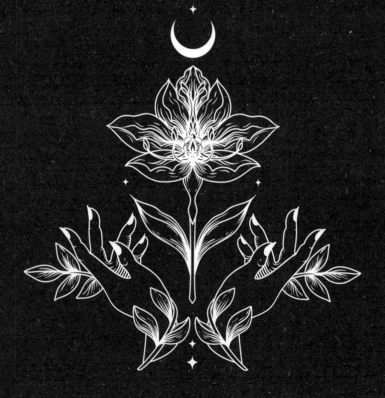

Introduction

ow that we've laid the foundation of working with the wombspace holistically, this section of the book will supply you with knowledge on herbs and holistic therapies to further support the body through every phase of life and the menstrual cycle. Here you will learn how to make herbal medicines and find suggested herbal recipes, remedies, and easy-to-use tools that will instill you with wisdom that has been used for centuries. Working with plants in this type of intimate way invites not only their healing capabilities, but also the magick they hold when used intentionally.

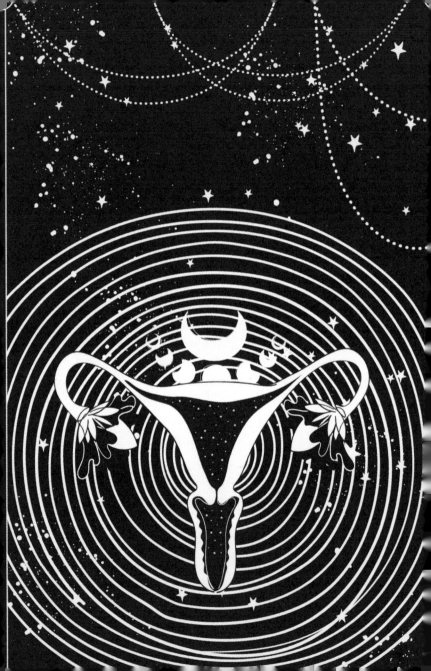

Chapter Seven: Herbal Recipes for Every Womb

*H*ere we begin the process of learning the folk methods of making herbal medicine. In the pages to come, I will cover medicine making with water, alcohol, honey, oil, and vinegar. Every section will offer instructions on how to make medicines with fresh or dry herbs. With honey and oil, you will find instructions for heated and non-heated methods. Note: these medicines may be made in varying ways. There are a variety of methods to learn, and what is overviewed here are simply the ones I choose to employ and teach. The equipment you will need for every medicine includes a clean jar, herb(s) of choice, menstruum, a label and writing utensil, and a piece of parchment paper for under the lid.

As you approach this material, my advice is to thoroughly read this information and think of a few medicines you want to make. Then, once you have ensured you've followed all of the safety instructions as reviewed in Chapter Six, make the medicines! You will learn best through the process of practice.

Most importantly, remember that this is a process of learning. And, to fail is to learn. Any "fails" in the plant medicine making world will only make you a stronger herbalist, and wiser when making an extraction the next time around. Take notes of your methods, be kind to yourself, and consider seeking out fellow budding herbalists as you learn.

Teas and Tisanes

Teas and tisanes are water extractions of herbs, which is how we make a medical extraction through combining plant material and water. A tea and a tisane are different things, depending on who you ask. Some folks consider tea to only be from *Camellia sinensis* varieties, which are traditional black and green teas. In that case, herbal teas would be referred to as tisanes. However, herbal teas and tisanes are the same thing. For simplicity's sake, I refer to them as teas.

A tea/tisane extracts the water-soluble compounds found in the flowers and leaves of the herb being used. To make a water extraction out of berries, barks, and roots, you will want to make a decoction, which we will review in the following section. Teas/tisanes are traditionally made with 1 teaspoon of dried herb per cup of hot water, steeped from 5 to 15 minutes, depending on the herb, with a lid atop of the container and then strained. The lid will ensure the aromatics and plant constituents remain in the tea and do not escape through the steam. If using fresh plant material, use three times the amount of plant material.

While you can use less or more of the desired plant material in teas, it is important to remain consistent with steep times. Aim to steep these water extractions for an average of 7 to 8 minutes and no longer than 10 to 15 minutes, unless using nourishing herbs, which we will review in the coming pages. For more delicate plant material, such as rose petals, opt for a shorter steep time.

Herbal Decoctions

For a water extraction of roots, barks, seeds, and sometimes berries, such as rose hips and hawthorne berries, it is best to make a decoction. These plant materials are more dense and require a longer extraction process, as opposed to the delicate nature of flowers and leaves, which require less heat and steep time to preserve their medicinal elements. A decoction involves brewing water and herbs on a stovetop for a set period of time.

To make a decoction:

Place 1 teaspoon to 1 tablespoon of plant material to every 2 cups of water into a small stovetop-safe pot. Allow plant material to sit in the water for 10 to 30 minutes; this step is not necessary, but will make for a better brew.

Over medium high heat, bring water to a light, steady simmer for 20 to 25 minutes, uncovered.

If you have over 4 cups of water, you may want to adjust your cook time as the aim is to simmer almost one-half of the water off of the top. Strain the plant material from the water and immediately use your decoction. Or, store in the fridge for 2 to 3 days.

Herbal Infusions

Regularly drinking herbal infusions will change your life for the better when you find the nourishing herb that supports your systems the best. I can anecdotally admit, with experience from my own life and countless others I have worked with, that herbal infusions have the ability to make your skin glow, your hair strong, and your energy more sustained, all signs of effective nourishment. These are the reasons why they are repeatedly recommended throughout the herbal portion of this book.

You may be wondering, "What is so different about these water extractions than the others?" Simply put, herbal infusions are long water extractions of specific plants called nourishing herbs, which are the only herbs that are safe to steep for a lengthy amount of time. Additionally, these infusions require a much higher volume of plant matter than what is used in teas.

Nourishing herbs are wild "weeds" full of vitamins, nutrients, enzymes, and minerals our bodies need to fully function at their best capacity. The plants included in this category are Dandelion Root/Leaf, Burdock Root, Chickweed, Cleavers, Red Clover, Red Raspberry Leaf, Nettle, Oatstraw/Milky Oat Tops, Marshmallow Root, Linden Leaf and Flower,

Hawthorne Berries/Leaves/Flowers, Violet Flower/Leaf, and Calendula. These plants share a commonality that they are nutrients, vitamin rich, and generally safe to use for most people. Where our foods leave nutritional gaps, herbal infusions come in to further nourish our bodies.

Many of the plants used for herbal infusions are considered food as they are as gentle as food, some of which are eaten whole. They gently cleanse, purify blood, remove toxins, and improve circulation, digestion, and elimination. They support our systems with such vigor that their nourishment is deep, reaching beyond the physical. Many find that the vitality provided by using plants in this way allows for their medicine to hold a profound capacity to hold space and allow for release in our emotional, mental, and spiritual bodies. When we are nourished on this level, it creates spaciousness, allowing us the energy required to move through emotions and feelings that may feel more dense when mental fogginess and vitality is low. With this, we are more able to find ease and joy in our days. A perfect example of "as above, so below."

To Make an Herbal Infusion

Place one heaping handful, or one ounce, of the nourishing herb(s) of your choice inside of a french press or a quart-sized mason jar. Top with hot water. If you will be using a root or dried berries, you'll want to decoct them first. Next, you will allow the herbs and water to macerate[79] for 6 to 12 hours, or overnight, before straining.

After you strain your infusion, you may make a second infusion with the plant material, as the plants will still contain some additional nutritional benefits. This can be done by following the same steps for the first infusion; however, you do not need to add more plant material. (While this infusion won't

---

79 Macerate refers to the extraction process of steeping herbs for a set period of times.

be as strong, it will give you the last bits of nutrients from your herbs.) After the second steeping, throw the herbs into compost.

Once your herbal infusion is finished, drink 2 to 4 cups of it daily. To receive the full benefits of daily infusions, aim for no less than 2 cups a day. Your infusion can be kept in the fridge for 1 to 3 days, depending on the herb you use. These extractions can be made as simples, which means that only one plant is used. However, they can also be combined. As you use these plants individually, you will learn which ones you feel called to combine and experiment with.

These infusions may be used for things other than drinking and may be employed topically as well.

Some examples:

- Nettle infusions work as an excellent hair rinse and are known to strengthen and promote shine, and they may help alleviate dandruff. Topically on skin, its properties are known to soothe a sunburn, rash, or insect stings.
- A cold infusion[80] of marshmallow root is great relief for dry skin, inflamed nipples from breastfeeding, or an infected wound.
- A linden infusion is a divine addition to a bath aromatically and promotes relaxation.

Herbal Tinctures

Tinctures are easy-to-use, ready-to-go medicines typically made with alcohol. These medicines extract the alcohol-soluble (which are also fat-soluble) compounds found in plants, mushrooms, and seeds. These medicines are shelf stable and can last up to 2 to 3 years with proper storage in a dark, cool place. In addition to being a convenient way to imbibe herbs, tinctures

---

80 A cold infusion is best used for bringing out the demulcent, cooling qualities of herbs, which would otherwise be destroyed by the heat process. Simply cover plant material with room temperature water instead of hot water and allow to steep for 2 to 8 hours.

allow for extracting compounds otherwise not available in water extractions and are an excellent way to imbibe plants that one may be averse to drinking as a tea. Tinctures can be used directly in the mouth or in water/soda/tea.

Commonly, you'll find alcohol-based tinctures are made with cane alcohol or vodka. However, you can also make tinctures with tequila, brandy, rum, gin, or any spirit with a proper alcohol-by-volume ratio. In order to achieve the proper strength needed to extract the plant medicine, my preference is to aim to achieve a 40 percent of alcohol by volume, or 80 proof. If using an alcohol with a higher proof of alcohol, it is important to dilute with water prior to creating an herbal medicine to bring the mixture to 80 to 90 proof. *Example: Combine 1 cup of distilled or spring water to one cup of 190 proof cane alcohol.*

Note: To make tinctures alcohol-free, use food grade glycerine. Glycerine tinctures are typically called glycerites.

How to Make an Herbal Tincture

Fresh Herbs
Tear or chop the herbs and pack the jar completely full with plant material, filling it to the lip of the jar, leaving around 1 to 1.5 inch space at the top. Top with alcohol of choice. Allow liquid to settle and air bubbles to release. Slowly continue to top off with alcohol until plant material is covered.

Dried Herbs
Fill jar one-half of the way full with dried plant material. Top with alcohol of choice. Allow liquid to settle and slowly top off with alcohol until plant material is covered.

For both methods, top the lid with a piece of parchment paper prior to placing on the lid. Shake the jar vigorously and label. Macerate this medicine for 4 to 6 weeks, or longer, shaking the jar daily or as frequently as you remember to do so. Strain, compost, and store the tincture in a cool, dark place.

Herbal Infused Honey

I have a true love for herbal infused honeys. They are delicious, are easy to make and forget about, and can be used in a series of delightful ways. To sweeten the deal, using raw honey offers a wide range of beneficial medicinal qualities which include antimicrobial, anti-inflammatory, and antioxidant elements.[81] Additionally, raw honey provides enzymes and amino acids for the digestive system, and some studies show there are prebiotics present as well.[82] As long as the moisture content is in balance, honey will suspend your favorite medicinal flower, plants, roots, and berries for a very long time, if not forever.

This bears repeating: excess moisture is the enemy of a plant medicine made with oil and honey. Don't use herbs you've harvested after a rainy day or dewey morning and don't wash your herbs before making medicine with them. Unless, of course, you have harvested muddy roots, which will need to be soaked, processed, and possibly dried.

Always consider if there is too much moisture content in the plant part you are trying to use. Plants with higher water content may include plants high in essential oils, flowers with many layers, roots, and plants that have condensation, dew, or water atop of them. Your medicine may benefit from allowing the plant material to wilt for one day prior to infusing them. However, some plant materials may not be well suited for a specific medicinal extraction or without the use of heat. Dandelion flowers are a good example of a plant that will more

---

81 "Honey and Health: A Review of Recent Clinical Research," *Pharmacognosy Research*, 2015, hero.epa.gov/hero/index.cfm/reference/details/reference_id/4243861.
82 "The Potential of Honey as a Prebiotic Food to Re-engineer the Gut Microbiome Toward a Healthy State," *Frontiers in Nutrition*, 2021, frontiersin.org/journals/nutrition/articles/10.3389/fnut.2022.957932/full.

than likely spoil your oil or honey medicine if used without heat, as they contain too much water content. Conversely, rose petals are delicate, are less water rich, and will typically be fine to use fresh.

Ways you can use herbal honeys:

- In tea: Simply scoop 1 teaspoon of herbal honey (unstrained or strained) and add to a hot cup of water. Stir. Strain if using unstrained honey.

- Does your recipe call for honey? Make it medicinal and use herbal honey. Baked goods. On pancakes. In granola bars. Marshmallows. Ice cream.

- Topically: On acne, blisters, sores, scrapes, burns, and bruises. Depending on what herb you've infused with your honey, chances are it could be brought in for skin healing. If using unstrained honey, ensure plant material does not enter an open wound.

- Syrups: Elderberry syrup for winter. Lavender syrup for homemade lemonade. There are endless options, and I will suggest some fun combinations in the Syrups section. Infused honey is a pathway to medicinal syrup.

- In other medicines: As we will learn in the vinegars section, you can infuse your medicinal honey with apple cider vinegar to make a range of delicious potions.

There are two ways to make herbal infused honey—with heat or without heat. While the heat method very gently raises the heat of the honey, I tend to veer towards using the non-heat method for my herbal infused honey medicines, unless the plant material requires heat, such as cannabis or a plant with a high water content. The non-heat method ensures the honey will remain raw. Above all, we want to avoid any air bubbles and moisture/water, as these situations are grounds for mold to grow.

Reminder: Be sure to put wax or parchment paper at the mouth of the jar before sealing it shut. Ensure plant material is submerged in the menstruum. Label your jars!

Herbal Infused Honey, Non-Heat Method

Fresh Herbs

Tear, or chop, your herbs. This allows for more surface area of the plant to be exposed, which will allow for a more potent medicine. Pack the jar completely full with plant material, filling it to the lip of the jar, leaving around a 1 to 1.5 inch space from the very top of the jar. Slowly top with honey. You'll want to allow the honey to sink down through the plant material to the bottom of the jar. Be sure to not overfill it. After gravity has pulled most of the honey down, use a chopstick, and stir to combine. This will also release air bubbles. Repeat this process until you are sure every part of the herbs are saturated in honey and there are no remaining air bubbles. You will want the herbs to be fully submerged in honey prior to placing a lid atop.

Dried Herbs

Fill your jar one-half of the way full with dried herbs. Slowly top with honey. Allow the honey to sink down through the plant material to the bottom of the jar. Be sure to not overfill. Using a chopstick, stir to combine. Repeat this process until all of the plant material is completely saturated in honey and there are no remaining air bubbles.

For both methods, macerate the herbs in the honey for 4 to 6 weeks, or longer, tipping the jar back and forth daily or every time you think of it. There is an option to strain the herbs from the honey, or allow them to remain submerged.

Straining herbs from honey can be a messy process. If you decide to do this, use cheesecloth or a fine mesh strainer. If using cheesecloth, place the cheesecloth inside of a funnel suspended at the top of a clean jar and slowly pour the honey into it. Pull all ends together in a bunch, and squeeze the honey from the herbs.

If you choose not to strain your honey, you can use the infused honey directly from the jar as needed.

Herbal Infused Honey, Heat Method

For the heated method, you will use the same measurements described in the non-heat method. There are two options here: stovetop and crockpot.

For the stovetop: Combine honey and herbs in a mason jar and pour its contents into a saucepan. Gently heat on medium and stir to combine. Once the mixture starts to bubble, take off heat immediately. Allow to completely cool. Repeat this process 4 times. On the fourth time, strain herbs from honey. Allow honey to cool before putting the lid on the jar. Be sure to label your medicine. Store honey in a cool, dark space.

For crockpot: Combine honey and herbs in a mason jar with a tightly sealed lid. Place into a crockpot and cover with water just under the lip of the jar. Place heat setting to warm. Macerate for 10 to 12 hours during the day, shaking the jar every 2 to 3 hours. Rest overnight. Repeat this process for 3 to 4 days. Strain or place the jar aside to store in a cool, dark place.

Note: If using a plant with a high water content, it is advisable to remove the lid during the maceration process. Use a wooden utensil to stir the contents of the jar during the extraction process.

Herbal Honey Making Inspiration

Use any single herbs, called simples, or combinations, to make some delightful herbal infused honeys. These are some of my favorites combinations:

- Rose and Tulsi: a blend that is relaxing and harmonic
- Goldenrod and Nettle: to be used before and during seasonal allergies
- Fresh Ginger Root and Turmeric: a warming digestive tonic
- Mint and Raspberries: a truly delicious summer medley

- Blueberries and Garden Sage: same as the above
- Simples: Forsythia Flowers, Rosehips, Violet Flower, Raspberry Leaf, Peppermint, Lemon Balm, Sage, Rosemary, Yarrow

Syrups

Herbal Syrups are an excellent and delicious way to incorporate herbs into your everyday life. This form of herbal medicine is a little bit easier to travel with and use on-the-go. Syrups make great additions to drinks, baked goods, salads, and marinades. And, for the people and kids in your life who may feel averse to taking herbal medicines, this can be a good way to introduce it into their lives.

Note: I use honey as my sweetener for these examples. You can also use cane sugar, agave, maple syrup, or any other sweetener of your choice.

Herbal Syrup Recipes

For Leaves, Bark, Roots, Berries, and Seeds
Make a decoction with 1 part herbs (fresh or dry) to 2 parts water.

Combine in saucepan, simmer until one-half of the water you started with remains.

Strain herbs and pour liquid back into saucepan.

Allow liquid to cool.

Add in 1 cup of honey to saucepan.

If necessary, gently heat, allowing the ingredients to just combine (to keep those raw enzymes in there).

Allow to cool and store in glass container in fridge.

To Make Syrup with Flowers
Use 4 parts flowers to 1 part water and 1 part honey.

Place flowers in a jar or bowl. Bring the water to a heavy simmer and pour on top. Cover with a lip and steep for 10 to 40 minutes, depending on how strong you want the syrup to be. Strain and stir in 1 part honey. Allow to cool and store in a glass container in the fridge.

These syrups will keep in the fridge for 1 to 2 months. However, if you add 1 part tincture or alcohol to 3 parts of syrup, you will extend the life up to 9 months!

If you want to make your syrups even more potently medicinal, I suggest using previously herbal infused honey.

Elderberry Syrup Recipe
- 1 cup (dried) elderberries
- 2 cups water
- 1 cup honey
- 1 Tablespoon Ceylon cinnamon
- 1 teaspoon clove, ground
- A pinch of cardamom

Cook on medium heat to simmer, mashing berries as it cooks. You will then have 1 cup of strong elderberry tea. Strain out berries from water.

Once cooled, add in clove, Ceylon cinnamon, and cardamom. Gently warm to combine. Allow to cool and add honey.

Optional: Add .5 cup and 2.5 tablespoons of elderberry tincture or brandy to syrup

Store in fridge!

Tinctures to combine with this syrup: Yarrow, Cleavers, Reishi, Turkey Tail, Violet.

Other Syrup Ideas
These are some of my personal favorite, most used, herbal syrup simples and combinations.
- Cherry Bark: used as a cough syrup

- Passionflower, Skullcap, Lemon Balm, and Catnip: sleepy time syrup
- Lilac and Cherry Juice: instead of water, use cherry juice
- Rose Flower and Cardamom: excellent in an herbal latte
- Elderberry Syrup Recipe, sweetened with Yarrow Infused Honey and Cleavers Tincture: makes an extra potent elderberry syrup
- Violet Flower: add a few drops of lemon to change the color

Pastilles

Pastilles are small herb and honey balls made with powdered herbs that act as soft lozenges. They travel easily, make less palatable herbs easier to take, and are a fun way to consume your medicine. If you have someone in your life who doesn't want to take their herbs but needs to, this may be the way to do it. Pastilles typically are made with 1 part honey to 3 part powdered herbs.

To make: Place powdered herbs in a small bowl and top with honey. Using a wooden spoon or chopstick, stir to combine. You will want a dough that will be easy to work with and isn't droopy. Add more powdered herbs if the mixture doesn't start to come into a thicker state when fully combined. Next, roll the dough into small, nickel sized balls. Once balls are formed, roll them in either the powdered herb you used, or a tastier one. If you were making pastilles out of a bitter herb, consider using something like cacao, cinnamon, licorice, or marshmallow root powder.

Place on cookie sheet and dry in the sun for 1 to 2 days or dehydrate

Store in a glass container.

Pastille Combinations
- Activated Charcoal and Bentonite Clay: excellent if you have exposure to mold, toxic environments, or experience

fire season. NOTE: For this combination, ONLY use wooden utensils or chopsticks to stir and combine

Digestive System Soothing Blends
- Turmeric and Black Pepper
- Ginger and Chamomile
- Marshmallow Root and Cinnamon
- Ginger, Turmeric, Clove, and Cardamom

Nervous System Support
- Rose and Tulsi
- Shatavari, Marshmallow Root, Rose, and Cinnamon
- Lemon Balm, Licorice Root, and Skullcap (NOTE: You will want only 5 percent of your powdered herb to consist of Licorice Root.)
- Ashwagandha, Cacao, and Cinnamon

Electuaries

Electuaries are similar to pastilles, but are made with much more honey and appear as a paste. You can choose how thick, or thin, you want this mixture to be.

The Formula
- 1 part powdered herb to 2 parts honey
- Stir to combine with a wooden chopstick and keep in a glass jar

Electuary Inspiration
- Golden Milk Blend (Turmeric, Black Pepper, and Ginger)
- Chai Latte Blend (Ceylon Cinnamon, Ginger, Cardamom, and Clove)
- Gut Heal Blend (Ginger, Marshmallow Root, and Licorice Root) (NOTE: You will want only 5 percent of your powdered herb to consist of licorice root.)
- Chocolate, Orange Dream (Orange Zest, Cacao, a pinch of Cardamom, and a splash of Vanilla)

- Adaptogenic[83] Powerhouse (Ashwagandha, Reishi Mushroom, Turkey Tail Mushroom, Tulsi, Cacao, and Cinnamon)
- Sunny Escape (Meyer Lemon Zest and Ginger)

Herbal Vinegars

How did I ever survive before I was taught how to make herbal-infused vinegars? My countertops, my salad dressings, and my poison oak rashes cannot recall. These magickal vinegars most commonly use apple cider vinegar as it is mineral rich, beneficial to digestion, toning to skin, and has been shown to reduce blood sugar spikes.[84] If you feel inspired to do so, you can opt to use other kinds of vinegar, such as balsamic or white vinegar.

An herbal infused vinegar can be used in any way you would traditionally use vinegar. In marinades, dressings, topically as a toner and/or to alleviate skin problems, in soda water, as a house cleaning spray. These extractions are simple to make and follow the same guidelines as herbal infused honeys.

A REMINDER: Be sure to put wax or parchment paper at the mouth of the jar before sealing your medicines shut. Vinegar will quickly corrode them. Ensure plant material is submerged in the menstruum. Label your jars!

Fresh Herbs

Tear, or chop herbs. This allows for more surface area of the plant to be exposed, which will allow for a more potent medicine. Pack the jar completely full with plant material, filling it to the lip of the jar, leaving around a 1 to 1.5 inch space from the very top of the jar. Top with vinegar. Allow to rest so that air bubbles

---

83 Adaptogenic refers to adaptogens, which are herbs that increase the body's response and resistance to stress.
84 "Beneficial Effects of Apple Vinegar on Hyperglycemia and Hyperlipidemia in Hypercaloric-Fed Rats," *Journal of Diabetics Research*, 2020, ncbi.nlm.nih.gov/pmc/articles/PMC7374219/.

can release. Top off with more vinegar until all plant material is submerged in vinegar, but do not overfill.

Dried Herbs

Fill your jar one-half of the way full with dried herbs. Slowly top with vinegar. Allow the honey to sink down through the plant material to the bottom of the jar. Be sure to not overfill it. Using a chopstick, stir to combine. Repeat this process until all of the plant material is completely saturated in honey and there are no remaining air bubbles.

For both of these methods, you will macerate the herbs in the vinegar for 4 to 6 weeks, or longer, shaking the jar daily or every time you remember to do so. When you wish to use your medicine, strain the herbs from the vinegar and pour into a clean vessel, making sure to label that jar.

Oxymels

Oxymels are a divine combination of honey, vinegar, and herbs. This elixir contains all of the medicinal qualities of honey and vinegar, which will offer a medicine that is rich in digestive system benefits, healthy bacteria, and antimicrobial and antibacterial properties. These potions are great to enjoy straight, in soda water as a mocktail or refreshing beverage, or to use as a dressing/marinade.

Standard Oxymel Recipe

The standard oxymel recipe is 1 part apple cider vinegar (ACV) to 1 part honey.

Fill the jar with herbs in the same way you would if you were making herbal honey or herbal vinegar. Reminder, this means the jar should be one-half full with dried herb, or pack plant material to the lip of the jar for fresh plant material. Pour one-half of the way full with ACV and top the other half with honey. Place wax paper on top of the mouth of the jar, following with the lid. Shake around vigorously. Check to ensure herbs are fully submerged.

Note, you can adjust the ratios here if you want the medicine to be more sweet or tangy.

Allow to macerate for 4 to 6 weeks, shaking the jar daily or every time you think to do so. Strain out herbs and pour back into the jar you used, or into a clean jar with a proper label. Use within 6 months and store in a dark, cool space.

My Favorite Oxymel Combinations
- Goldenrod, Nettle, and Elderberry (allergy relief and tonic)
- Rose (as a simple)
- Lemon Balm and Clary Sage (calming and clarity)
- Nettle (a simple) (great not only internally, but topically and for hair too)
- Rosemary, Sage, and Thyme (excellent marinade and dressing)
- Peppermint (a simple) (for soothing digestive upset)

Shrubs

Shrubs are similar to oxymels, but involve a fermentation process. They are a bit more labor intensive, but are ready to use in just 2 weeks. If you like kombucha, jun, or any other fermented bubbly drinks, there is a high likelihood you'll absolutely love shrubs. Shrubs traditionally involve a mixture of vinegar, honey, fruits, herbs, and juice. If you want to make the medicine of a plant taste better, consider incorporating it into a shrub. Due to their fermentation process, they act as a digestive tonic, will aid in alleviating allergies, are antimicrobial, and contain live cultures that are known to have cancer-protective properties.

A Standard Shrub Recipe
- Apple cider vinegar
- Fruit/juicier roots/berries

- Aromatic herbs
- Juice (such as lemon/lime/orange)
- Honey
- Cheesecloth or breathable, natural fabric

Fill mason jar one-half full of fruit/roots/berries. Muddle them to release aromas and juices. Place any aromatic herbs on top. Cover with ACV, allowing for 1 inch of space from the top of the jar. Ensure ingredients are submerged in vinegar. Drape cheesecloth over the lid and leave the jar in a dark, undisturbed place for 12 hours.

After 12 hours, replace the cheesecloth with parchment/wax paper and place the lid on the jar. Over the course of 3 days, shake the jar as often as you remember to, being sure to store the jar remains in a dark, cool place.

After 3 days have passed, strain the contents of the jar from the vinegar. Carefully pick out any of the aromatic herb material and discard. Place the fruit/berry/root materials back into the jar and shake to combine. Store the jar in the fridge for 4 more days and shake often.

Strain all plant material from vinegar. Depending on how much liquid you have, you may want to pour the vinegar in a bigger jar as you will want to have one-half of a jar full of the infused vinegar. Fill one-fourth more of the way full with juice of choice, and the remainder one-fourth with honey. Shake to combine. Allow to sit in the fridge for 1 more week before using.

Keep refrigerated.

Enjoy with soda water, as a mocktail, straight, or in any other way you feel pulled to use this delicious concoction.

Delicious Shrub Blends
- Lilac Flowers, Lemon Juice, and Strawberries (an instantly uplifting combination)
- Lemon, Ginger, and Rosemary Sprigs (digestive system love)

- Ginger, Turmeric, Orange Juice, and a touch of Black Pepper (more digestive system support)
- Nectarine, Red Beet, and Goldenrod Flowers (a happy, blood-building tonic)
- Blackberry, Cherry Juice, and Sage (aromatic, digestive system support)
- Blood Orange and Rosemary (delicious)

Herbal Oils

The methods for herbal infused oils discussed here are for topical use. Our skin is the largest organ on our body, which makes these medicines a wonderful way to receive a plant's medicinal benefits. Oils typically used for these extractions include extra virgin olive oil, avocado oil, safflower oil, sunflower oil, sesame oil, castor oil, jojoba oil, shea butter, cocoa butter, and coconut oil. Each oil has varying medicinal qualities within itself and will combine differently with beeswax when making salves and other potions. Keep in mind that when creating an extraction with oils/fats that are solid at room temperature, like coconut oil and shea butter, the heat method must be utilized.

Herbal infused oils can be turned into salves, soaps, lotions, and creams. They are also excellent on their own. I encourage you to use these extractions in the form of oil before moving on to making other things with them, as this will allow you to register the scope of their medicinal and spiritual qualities.

REMINDER: Be sure to put wax or parchment paper at the mouth of the jar before sealing your medicines shut. Ensure plant material is submerged in the menstruum. Label your jars!

To get started, you will need a jar, oil of choice, and your herb(s) of choice.

Non-Heat Method with Fresh Herbs

You will need to carefully decide if the plant(s) you are using are suitable for using fresh in the non-heat method. Plants that contain a low amount of moisture are the best candidates for the non-heat method. Examples of these are lavender, cedar leaves, rosemary, oregano leaf, or sage. If the plant you are looking to use has a higher water content, and you are looking to use this method, I suggest allowing the plant material to wilt for one to two days prior to infusing it in oil.

Tear, or chop, your herbs. This allows for more surface area of the plant to be exposed, which will allow for a more potent medicine. Pack a jar completely full with plant material, filling it to the lip of the jar, leaving around a 1 to 1.5 inch space from the very top of the jar. Top with oil. Using a wooden chopstick, poke through the oil and plant mixture to release any air bubbles and to fully coat plant material. Repeat as needed. Ensure that all plant material is submerged in oil. Unlike the rest of the medicines we've learned how to make in this guidebook, you will want to fill it with oil to the very top of the jar.

Non-Heat Method with Dried Herbs

Fill the jar one-half of the way full with dried herb. Top with oil. Using a wooden chopstick, poke through the oil and plant mixture to release any air bubbles and to fully coat plant material. Repeat as needed. Ensure that all plant material is submerged in oil. Unlike the rest of the medicines we've learned how to make in this guidebook, you will want to fill it with oil to the very top of the jar.

For both of these methods, you will macerate the herbs in the oil for 4 to 6 weeks, and no longer. Shake the jar daily or as often as you remember to do so. The plant material will absorb the oil as time goes on. You will need to check it regularly and top off with oil as needed. It is wise to keep the jar on a towel (that you don't mind ruining), as oil tends to seep from the lid as this process unfolds. Place the jar out of sunlight. However, this mixture can stand to be in a warmer storage space. After decanting your mixture, store your herbal infused oil in a clean glass jar. Your oil has the potential to last for years if you also keep it refrigerated.

Heat Method

For the heated method, you will use the same ratios described in the non-heat method. For heat, choose between using a crockpot or stovetop.

Combine oil and plant material in a mason jar. Place the jar in the pot or crockpot and fill with water, just to the lip of the jar. If using a crockpot, turn to the warm setting. If using a stovetop, place the saucepan on the lowest heat setting. Shake the jar every few hours. Macerate for 2 to 3 days. If using a stovetop, consider turning off the heat when you're asleep and turning back on when you awake.

To decant, place cheesecloth in a large funnel and place into a clean jar. Pour contents of the infusion into cheesecloth and strain, squeezing cheesecloth clean of oil. Allow to settle for 24 hours. Plant material will settle at the bottom of the jar. Slowly pour off herbal infused oil into another clean jar, being careful to not get sediment into the jar. Keep stored out of light in a cool, dark place. As long as moisture remains out of this oil, it can last up to years if stored in the refrigerator.

Salves

If you've ever had a scrape, blister, burn, bee sting, splinter, or skin malady that needed some TLC, you've been a person who could use a salve. While oils are best for when you want the medicine to deeply penetrate your body's tissues, salves remain at the surface, tending to the healing of wounds and other skin maladies where you want to avoid infection and bring in deep nourishment.

Salves are made by melting beeswax into herbal infused oils. The finished product will depend on how thick you wish to make the ointment.

To start, use 1 part beeswax to 5 parts oil. Slowly combine them in a saucepan, or double boiler, on low heat, stirring frequently until the beeswax is completely melted. To test the consistency of the oil, pour a small amount of the oil into a metal spoon and place in the freezer. This is called the "spoon test." Wait for around 1 to 2 minutes. Use the ointment to see if it is the consistency you wish for. If it is too hard, add more oil. If it is too soft, add more beeswax. Repeat the spoon test until you have reached your desired consistency.

Immediately pour the mixture into jars. Completely cool before placing lids on jars and labeling.

My Most Cherished Herbal Oils and Salve Combinations

- An all-purpose salve can be made with any (or all, or a combination) of the following: Chickweed, Nettle, Violet Leaf, Cleavers, Plantain Leaf, and Calendula.
- Cedar and Hemlock Tree Leaf (excellent musculoskeletal, relaxing body oil)
- Violet and Rose Flower (womb and breast massage salve)
- Lavender and Mugwort (a reproductive system support during menstruation)
- Mugwort and Ginger (for painful, stagnant periods)
- Blue Lotus, Passionflower, Damiana, and Mugwort (ritual, dreamspace ointment)

Chapter Eight: Herbalism & Holistic Therapies for Every Menstrual Phase

*T*he main priority during menstruating years should be simply this: supportive, holistic nourishment. As our bodies enact the menstrual cycle during our reproductive years, hormones are fluctuating, blood is regularly being lost, and our nutrient needs are great. There are herbs, nutritional supplements, and holistic practices which we can use to nourish and support our bodies during this time, in addition to using the foods discussed previously.

Nourishing herbs and culinary herbs can sweep in to bring in a bounty of minerals, vitamins, and overall support to the body systems that are hard at work. Here, we will review deeply restorative supportive herbs for each phase of the menstrual cycle. For these suggestions, we focus on using these plants as herbal infusions, which as discussed in the previous chapter, are water extractions which are steeped for 6 to 8 hours. These infusions allow for the highest mineral and vitamin concentrations in bioavailable forms and encourage overall lymph movement. In this section of the book, I refrain from addressing herbs that are supportive to other menstrual conditions that may arise. You may locate that information in Chapter 10.

The supplements I'll share for each phase are basic vitamins and minerals recommended by many health practitioners at the standard daily allowance for a healthy functioning body. You may feel called to implement one, some, or none of these supplements into your life. They are merely suggestions and information to know and consider.

After going through the phases and corresponding herb recommendations, I'll also be sharing holistic practices for the menstrual cycle. These suggestions contain some things which are applicable and helpful for all or varying seasons and stages of life. Even if you are not currently in your reproductive years, I highly suggest reading this section to glean what may be supportive to you or someone you know.

SAFETY NOTE: While the majority of these herbs, supplements, and practices are safe for most people, it is essential for you to do your homework to ensure they are not contraindicated for a health condition, a prescription pill, or if you are pregnant or trying to become pregnant. Please consult your healthcare provider or a clinically trained herbalist if you are unsure if something is right for you.

Herbs and the Menstrual Phase

The menstrual/early follicular phase's key herbal allies are **nettle leaf** (*Urtica dioica*) and **red raspberry leaf** (*Rubus idaeus*), due to their deeply nourishing compositions. Nettle leaf is a blood-building herb rich in magnesium, iron, zinc, and vitamins C, D, and K, which is what gives it its restorative embodiment. When bleeding during the menstrual phase, these are the nutrients and vitamins which need to be replenished in the body. This ensures that the body is properly prepared for the phases that follow for the remainder of your cycle.

As nettle is a diuretic, it is drying in nature and moves fluids from the body. This movement encourages waste removal and enhances the detoxification process: a supremely important assist in hormonal cell waste elimination.

Raspberry leaf is an herb mentioned often when it comes to female reproductive health as it works deeply to restore and bring health to the uterine lining and is antispasmodic in nature. The active compound in raspberry leaf, fragarine, aids in reducing menstrual cramps by relaxing the smooth muscles of the uterus. Like nettle leaf, raspberry leaf is full of minerals and vitamins such as magnesium, zinc, potassium, and iron. Raspberry leaf is most effective when used a few days prior to when you start bleeding, but has also been known to be effective if used acutely.

Consider drinking one quart of nettle, raspberry leaf, or a combined infusion of the two daily during this phase of your cycle. These long water extractions will pull the highest amount of minerals and vitamins and will hydrate you more deeply. As nettle leaf and raspberry leaf are energetically cooling and drying, some modifications may be needed for these infusions.

For folks that tend to run dry, consider adding a pinch of **marshmallow root** (*Althaea officinalis*) into the infusion after it has cooled. Marshmallow root is a mucilaginous, moistening herb that will assist in balancing the infusion. These moistening properties are preserved when used with room temperature water, as they are mostly destroyed with heat. For folks who tend towards a cold body composition, combine one part nettle leaf or raspberry leaf infusion with one part ginger root decoction. Continue steeping overnight or for 6 to 8 hours.

SAFETY NOTE: Nettle may be contraindicated for folks who are experiencing edema due to impaired cardiac or renal function.

Culinary Herbs to Incorporate

Turmeric, ginger, cinnamon, parsley, and cilantro are all herbs that have anti-inflammatory, nutritive qualities that will be of aid to the body while bleeding. These herbs incorporate well into meals, but can also be made into teas.

If using roots for a tea, like turmeric or ginger, you will need to decoct them.

Turmeric (*Curcuma longa*), when combined with a small pinch of black pepper, is known to soothe the mucous membranes of the stomach, which has a tendency of being sensitive during this phase.

Ginger (*Zingiber officinale*) is warming and carminative and also encourages healthy blood flow. As digestion is more prone to being negatively affected during the menstrual phase, ginger's actions may be a helpful presence for healthy digestion and assimilation of food. This may also be a wise choice to use if cramping is present, as it will bring warmth and blood flow to the womb space.

Ceylon cinnamon (*Cinnamomum verum*), like turmeric, is soothing to mucous membranes and aids in curbing overall inflammation. It is also known to effectively quell any nausea that may come with bleeding. Its energetics are warming and can also be moistening when extracted in room temperature water as a tea for at least 2 to 3 hours.

Parsley (*Petroselinum crispum*) is rich in antioxidants and Vitamins A, C, and K. It is also an emmenagogue, which is an herb that stimulates and encourages the menstrual flow. As it is ideal to keep blood flow at a consistent, thorough pace during menstruation, parsley may come in hand for those who experience scanty or slow to start periods.

Herbs and the Follicular Phase

Similar to the menstrual phase, nettle leaf will be of great aid during the follicular phase. Its diuretic and alterative qualities flushes the system of cell waste, including hormones which have been used by the body and need to be eliminated to prevent reabsorption. Nettle is also helpful in supplying the body with the nutrients it needs to start the process of releasing the egg for ovulation. As the body will still be in the process of regeneration from the blood lost during menstruation, nettle's iron-rich contents will help replenish the iron lost through menstrual blood during this time, which will also help ensure the production of red blood cells

Consider drinking one quart of nettle leaf infusions daily during the follicular phase alongside an adequate amount of fresh water throughout the day.

Due to high levels of hormone processing during the follicular phase, the body can tend towards dehydration. Infusions will not only provide you with water, but also with needed minerals and vitamins.

Herbs and the Ovulatory Phase

During the ovulatory phase, **dandelion root** (*Taraxacum officinalis*) and **calendula** (*Calendula officinalis*) infusions may be most supportive. Dandelion root is known to cleanse and clear the liver of excess hormones and build-up. It is cooling, bitter, and dry. As this plant aids in balancing blood-sugar levels, it can help avoid excessive sugar cravings, which are common during ovulation and hormone shifts. For bodies that run energetically cold, consider combining dandelion root and ginger root. These combine well together and create a synergistic effect energetically and are supportive allies to the digestive system.

While many think of calendula for topical wound healing, its golden blooms offer internal lymphatic qualities that offer cleansing and detoxifying elements to the whole body system. A 2022 study has shown that calendula extract use is supportive to ovulation as well as the promotion of the development of follicles.[85]

SAFETY NOTE: Dandelion root may be contraindicated for those who are taking prescription medications that include

---

85 "The Effect of Hydroalcoholic Calendula Officinalis Extract on Androgen-Induced Polycystic Ovary Syndrome Model in Female Rat," *BioMed Research International*, 2022.

water pills, blood thinners, lithium, antibiotics, or heart/blood pressure medications.

Herbs and the Luteal Phase

During the luteal phase, the body is flooded with hormones. Combined with unavoidable environmental factors, supporting our livers as much as we can is important for an efficient detoxification process. For this, **burdock root** (*Arctium lappa*) is incredibly supportive during this time. Burdock is an incredible blood cleanser, is protective to the liver, and aids in flushing out excess hormones. It is also a mild diuretic and nourishing tonic which contains prebiotic inulin, a great food for healthy gut bacteria. If skin conditions worsen during this time in your cycle, or if PMS acne is an issue, burdock may be a great ally to incorporate into your life as it is known to bring vibrancy to the skin and hair. Consider using it as a daily infusion or incorporate it into your meals during this phase.

Ginger root (*Zingiber officinale*) will likely be supportive during the luteal phase. Ginger is warming, is an aid to digestion, and can ease bloating that may be present at this time. Ginger pairs well with **chamomile** (*Matricaria chamomilla*), which is known to ease anxious tension and digestive upset related to anxiety. For this, a decoction of ginger with a pinch of chamomile may be helpful.

Supplements Worth Using throughout the Menstrual Cycle

In an ideal world, we would be able to eat freshly prepared meals for every meal. However, even if we could eat entirely fresh foods, the reality is they are oftentimes lacking in the proper nutrition needed for our bodies thanks to environmental factors like depleted soil.

Luckily, we have supplements available to provide vital nutrients and minerals essential to our diets. I'm not one to advise others to depend on them as their sole source of nutrition, but I think that they are a good option to augment one's diet to prevent deficiencies. The vitamins listed below are ones highly recommended for most people. The dosage suggestions offered are a standard recommendation given by many health practitioners. However, do note that true needs may vary greatly from person to person. While I do not offer brand suggestions, it is necessary to mention that the quality of your supplements do matter. Higher price does not always equate to higher quality. So, how do you know if what you are buying is quality? Research the brand of supplements you are looking to use and find out if there have been third party tests done and published. Find a publication or someone that specializes in nutrition and see what supplements they recommend.

Vitamin D3

Vitamin D3 is a fat-soluble steroid hormone that boosts immunity, reduces inflammation, and may reduce period pain.[86] Food sources high in Vitamin D3 include fattier fish and fish liver oil. To receive adequate Vitamin D from the outdoors, aim for moderate sun exposure for 10 to 30 minutes a day without sunscreen,[87] slowly building up to that timeframe to avoid sunburn. During the winter months when the sun's rays are not strong enough to deliver proper Vitamin D, consider taking a supplement. It is essential that the supplement you take includes a fat source, such as an oil, or is taken with a fat source to ensure it is made bioavailable for the body.

Dosage: 2,000 IU a day[88]

86 "Office of Dietary Supplements - Vitamin D," n.d., ods.od.nih.gov/factsheets/VitaminD-HealthProfessional/.

87 "Vitamin D: Do We Need More Than Sunshine?", *American Journal of Lifestyle Medicine*, 2021 ncbi.nlm.nih.gov/pmc/articles/PMC8299926/.

88 Pludowski, P., Grant, W. B., Karras, S. N., Zittermann, A., & Pilz, S, "Vitamin D Supplementation: A Review of the Evidence Arguing for a Daily Dose of 2000

Magnesium

Magnesium is responsible for over 300 processes in the body including regulating muscle and nerve function, assisting in proper sleep, supporting the immune system, and maintaining energy production.[89] Dark chocolate, pumpkin seeds, bananas, beans, and avocados are food sources rich in magnesium.[90] While there are many different types of magnesium to supplement with, magnesium glycinate and magnesium citrate are two which are most commonly recommended.

Dosage: 300 to 400 mg per day.[91]

Zinc

Zinc is a trace mineral which plays a key role in the production of DNA and is greatly needed during times of growth such as puberty and pregnancy.[92] Zinc reduces inflammation, improves immunity, assists in regular development of eggs for ovulation, and is responsible for almost 100 enzymes to carry out imperative chemical reactions.[93] Food sources of zinc include oysters, seafood, nuts, and meat/poultry.[94]

Dosage: 8 to 12 mg a day

International Units (50 µg) of Vitamin D for Adults` in the General Population," *Nutrients* 16, 391, (2024), doi.org/10.3390/nu16030391

89 "Magnesium in Diet: MedlinePlus Medical Encyclopedia," n.d., medlineplus.gov/ency/article/002423.htm.

90 "25 Magnesium-Rich foods You Should Be Eating," Cleveland Clinic, June 27, 2024, health.clevelandclinic.org/foods-that-are-high-in-magnesium

91 Magnesium Supplement (Oral Route)," July 8, 2024, mayoclinic.org/drugs-supplements/magnesium-supplement-oral-route/proper-use/drg-20070730.

92 N. Roohani, R. Hurrell, R. Kelishadi, and R. Schulin, "Zinc and Its Importance for Human Health: An Integrative Review," PubMed Central (PMC), February 1, 2013, ncbi.nlm.nih.gov/pmc/articles/PMC3724376/.

93 "Zinc," The Nutrition Source, March 7, 2023, hsph.harvard.edu/nutritionsource/zinc/.

94 "Zinc," Office of Dietary Supplements, n.d., ods.od.nih.gov/factsheets/Zinc-HealthProfessional/.

B-Vitamins

B-Vitamins are water soluble vitamins which play important roles in the metabolic process, support healthy brain function, and maintain healthy skin cells.[95] They assist in regulating appetite, energy levels, and nervous system function.[96] Foods rich in B vitamins include meat (including liver), dark leafy greens, eggs, and seafood.

Dosage: Varies per brand

Omega-3s

Omega-3s are a group of fatty acids that contain ALA, EPA, and DHA. These fatty acids are essential to healthy brain and heart health, decrease overall inflammation, support bone density and health, and can help alleviate menstrual cramping symptoms.[97] Foods rich in Omega-3s include cold water fish such as salmon, tuna, sardines, and herring; nuts and seeds; and dark, leafy greens.

Dosage: 1 to 3 grams per day[98]

Holistic Modalities to Nourish the Body throughout the Menstrual Cycle

As we become more in touch with our menstrual cycles, it is important to get comfortable with our bodies as a whole. This involves looking at, touching, and tending to our bodies in ways that may be new to us.

---

95 M. Hanna, E. Jaqua, V. Nguyen, J. Clay, "B Vitamins: Functions and Uses in Medicine," *The Permanente Journal* 26, 89–97, (2022), doi.org/10.7812/tpp/21.204.
96 C. A. Calderón-Ospina and M. O. Nava-Mesa, "B Vitamins in the Nervous System: Current Knowledge of the Biochemical Modes of Action and Synergies of Thiamine, Pyridoxine, and Cobalamin," *CNS Neuroscience & Therapeutics*, 26, 5–13, (2019), doi.org/10.1111/cns.13207.
97 "Omega-3 Fatty Acids," Office of Dietary Supplements, n.d., ods.od.nih.gov/factsheets/Omega3FattyAcids-HealthProfessional/.
98 Ask Huberman Lab. (n.d.). Ask Huberman Lab. ai.hubermanlab.com/s/ZV-8W7Wc.

Here we will talk about a few practices that are reasonably accessible. Some require nothing but a bit of time, and some others call for a tool or two, but none of them involving a high price tag.

All of these practices involve awareness and circulation, two essential aspects to our reproductive health. Stimulating movement in these areas will optimize the lymphatic system. The lymph system moves our fluids throughout and out of the body, bringing flow to stagnate areas. A healthy lymph system promotes overall health. To support this, I challenge you to choose at least one of the following practices to implement regularly. Or, create your own practices that meet similar goals.

Breast and Womb Massage

Tight pants. Bras. Belts. Spandex. These things constrict the flow of fluids and blood that naturally occurs in our bodies when left to their own devices, sans tight materials.

So, how do we quell the issues that arise from these restrictive clothing items? Through routine, daily breast and womb-space massages. Whether you wear skinny jeans and bras or not, this is a practice that will create optimal health and much-needed circulation in these areas.

These self-massages offer countless benefits that include keeping multiple layers of the breast and womb tissue healthy; assisting in lymphatic flow movement; bringing deeper and more immediate awareness of any changes that may occur in either space; and cultivating a more in-tuned connection with yourself. Studies have shown that the squeezing and moving of the breast tissues can guide breast cancer cells into a normal growth pattern.[99]

99 "To Revert Breast Cancer Cells, Give Them the Squeeze," Berkeley, December 17, 2012, news.berkeley.edu/2012/12/17/malignant-breast-cells-grow-normally-when-compressed.

I find it easiest to incorporate this practice into my before or after showering/bathing, or before bedtime.

To start, apply a small amount of oil or salve to breasts. Pressing lightly but firmly, move counterclockwise with your hands, starting at the base of your breast and moving towards the nipple. Gently massage this area, feeling and taking note of every bump, node and tissue that surrounds and makes up your breasts. Repeat the same procedure in wombspace right below your belly button where your ovaries are. Over time, you'll intuitively figure out what works and feels best for you. As you start, pay close attention to what you feel and what feels tender, whether that is physically or emotionally.

If you are able to use an infused oil or salve made specifically for breast/womb massage, that's great. Plants that have an affinity for our lymphatic systems medicinally and spiritually include violet flower/leaf, rose petal, calendula, hawthorn blossoms, and red clover flower. However, organic olive oil, coconut oil, safflower, or hemp oil will work as well.

Moxibustion

Moxibustion, or moxa, is traditionally used in Traditional Chinese Medicine in tandem with acupuncture. Moxa consists of burning mugwort leaves (Artemis vulgaris), typically in the form of rolls, over areas/points where energy is cold, stagnant, inflamed, sore, "damp," painful, or in need of stimulation. In this application, mugwort is a friend to the womb. This plant has been historically used in many cultures for menstrual irregularities through stimulating blood flow, encouraging menstruation, and bringing relief to menstrual cramping. Moxa may be a great therapy to implement for relief of discomfort for painful periods, slow to start bleeding during menstruation, constipation related to PMS/menstrual phase, and for overall support in the wombspace if the body tends to run cold.

There are a handful of ways to practice this therapy, but for the sake of safety and also simplicity, we will be focusing on indirect moxibustion, where the lit moxa stick is held 1 to 2 inches over the body part where it is being applied.

I highly suggest finding a partner to administer this therapy for you so that you can fully relax, although it is possible to perform it on oneself. However, if the area you wish to work on isn't safe for you to personally do, DO NOT attempt to do this as you can severely burn yourself.

To use a moxa stick, light the end on fire until a coal forms. Carefully place the stick 1 to 2 inches above the area. Use slow, circular motions to distribute the heat through the area and to encourage blood flow. If you are concerned about the potential of getting burned, stick your pinky finger out as a stand to prevent getting burned. Do this for 3 to 5 minutes and take a break. Repeat for up to 10 to 15 minutes. Be sure to tap the end of the moxa stick into a heat safe container to rid it of its ashes in between applications. When putting out the stick, make sure it is fully extinguished.

As always, try everything at your own risk and after doing your own research for your own body. Not every method is for everybody. If you are pregnant or trying to become pregnant, do not use moxibustion unless under the guidance of a healthcare provider.

Castor Oil Packs

Castor oil packs. Maybe you've heard of them. Maybe you've tried them. Maybe none of this is true and you're thinking, "What the hell is a castor oil pack?" Let's do a quick breakdown.

Castor oil comes from the castor bean (Riconus communis) and contains a deep wealth of healing properties that include being:

- extremely calming to the nervous system,

- detoxifying to the tissues it's placed on,
- an alleviator of discomfort and stagnation,
- a lymphatic tool for circulation, restorative to damaged or scarred tissue

Castor oil packs over the wombspace may aid greatly when scar tissue, fibroids, ovarian cysts, or congestion of menses is involved. There are two ways to do a castor oil pack: with a heat source or as an overnight pack.

For both of these methods, I recommend designating an old outfit you don't care about to be your "castor oil pack outfit." The oil is thick, can be messy, and will put oil stains on clothes.

NOTE: Castor oil packs are not to be used every single day. At a maximum, it's recommended to do them 3-4 days a week. As you want to have rest days when working out intensely, our bodies need to have rest days when using detoxifying tools such as this. It is recommended to forego castor oil packs when you are bleeding as your body is in the depths of hard work and release.

Method #1

You'll need:
- Organic, cold-pressed castor oil
- A clean cloth and hand towel
- A heat source (heating pad or water bottle with hot water)
- A place to relax
- Pillows for propping legs

Prepare the space you will be relaxing in. Soak the clean cloth in castor oil so that it is drenched in oil. Place it directly on the area of choice. For womb supportive castor oil packs, place over uterus/ovaries. Lay down face up with legs propped up. Place a towel atop of the pack and place the heat source on top of that. Relax for at least 1 hour and up to 8 hours, or overnight. When finished. Wash the oil off of the skin and wash the cloth before using again.

Method #2

Right before going to bed, put on your castor oil pack outfit. Rub a thick layer of castor oil into the area so that you have a visible layer of castor oil. Be sure to wash the oil from the skin in the morning.

Body Scanning and Breathwork

Attuning yourself to your body bridges the connection between mind and body. This awareness awakens the inner knowing that no other person or practitioner can truly access. When we take the time to settle in and learn the inner workings of our physical state, we can more readily see how our mental, emotional, and spiritual sides influence our health.

Body scanning and breathwork are commonly associated with meditation and yoga. However, we will review ways to incorporate these methods and practices independent of meditation and yoga.

The examples highlighted in this section are introductory in nature. They can be practiced in the car, in bed before sleep, or before/during/after any moment where you become overwhelmed and need to find balance and calm.

Body Scanning

Body scanning involves bringing awareness to the body so that you can take note of where you feel tension, tightness, exhaustion, or stagnant energy.

If you experience menstrual-related symptoms/diseases/imbalances, this may be a good practice for you to tune into on a regular basis throughout your cycle. Take note of where you feel discomfort/tension/stagnation and what phase of your cycle you are in. This may better inform you in finding the root cause of these imbalances.

To begin, find a nice, quiet space to lie down or sit cross-legged. Relax into your position while also ensuring that the spine is straight. Close your eyes and steady your breath. Arrive in the moment. Start by envisioning and focusing on the very top of your head: the crown. Place all of your attention here. Breathe. Notice if there is any tension, pressure, aches, or pains. Once you feel you have fully perceived this area, slowly move down, doing the same with each and every inch of your body.

When you notice any disturbances/imbalances in an area, breathe into that space. Imagine that you are sending your breath to this specific area. Imagine your breath traveling from your lungs to this space. Hold the mental image of light and embodiment of healing to this space.

Remember to relax while doing this: Unclench your jar. Remove your tongue from the roof of your mouth. Let your shoulders slide towards the Earth. This should be a gentle practice. Try and stay with this process until you find a shift happens. If it doesn't, move on and take note of that area for the next time you do a body scan or practice breathwork.

Breathwork

Breathwork involves bringing awareness to your breath and steadying it through conscious effort and intention. This practice activates the parasympathetic nervous system, which slows our heart rate, promotes digestion and internal harmony, and lowers blood pressure.[100]

There is a wide range of ways to practice breathwork, ranging from dedicated classes and consultations and varying techniques you can try at home. In yoga, breathwork is referred to as pranayama.

Here we will review two easy-to-implement breathwork practices: square breathing and alternate nostril breathing

---

100 "Breathwork for beginners: What to Know and How to Get Started," July 24, 2024, Cleveland Clinic, health.clevelandclinic.org/breathwork.

Square breathing is a great technique to practice if you are experiencing anxiety, having difficulty falling asleep, or feeling tense/nervous for any number of reasons.

To practice this method, breathe in slowly through your nose for 5 counts. Then, hold your breath to the count of 5. Next, breathe out slowly through your mouth to the count of 5. And finally, hold your breath to the count of 5. Repeat this 4 times. Some find it helpful to imagine each inhale and exhale as a line that connects and extends from each other to create a square, hence the name square breathing.

Alternate nostril breathing is a yogic-based practice which involves breathing through one nostril at a time. Move into a comfortable seated position. Raise the right hand and stick out the pinky and thumb and bring towards your nose. Press the thumb against the right nostril, blocking it from air. And, inhale through the left nostril, slowly and steadily. When you have completed inhaling, lift your thumb, then press the pinky against the left nostril, blocking its air path. Exhale slowly and steadily through the right nostril. Continue to inhale through the right nostril. Then, block the right nostril and exhale through the left. Inhale through the left and repeat for two minutes, or until you feel a calm presence wash over you.

Chapter Nine: Herbalism & Holistic Therapies for the Womb Life Cycle: Maiden, Mother, Crone

*A*s we enter each phase of life, we enter new parts of ourselves: new stories that must be navigated emotionally, physically, and spiritually. Herbs offer us gentle guidance. They not only support all of the systems in our bodies, but also help ground us energetically, providing the necessary space needed to process the changes that come with entering a new phase of life.

Here we continue our discussion within the framework of Maiden, Mother, Crone through learning about herbs and holistic practices which are supportive through puberty to motherhood/parenthood and postpartum to menopause. As with much of this book, there is content to glean from each section which may be applied to related issues. These herbs and practices do not exist in a vacuum and offer a wide range of applications far beyond the scope discussed in these pages. Because of this, I highly recommend reading this chapter in its entirety, whether or not you believe this information pertains to you. The plants know no age, no gender, no bounds to which their wisdom can be applied. You will notice that the same herbs show up frequently. While there are no shortages of varying herbal medicines to use, my hope is that this exemplifies how multifaceted and highly dynamic each herb is. To know greatly about a few herbs is more powerful than knowing a little about many herbs.

Maiden: Applicable Herbs for Puberty

As discussed in the overview of our maiden phase in Chapter Three, puberty is a time of continuous transformation. The body, the psyche, and hormones are in flux, changing at the greatest rate our bodies will experience in our lives. In this section, we will explore herbs that can support and nourish various body systems, as well as emotional states experienced during this time.

SAFETY NOTES: Herb and drug contraindications are always important to consider prior to applying herbs to a body. It is important to ensure the herb you are taking will not negatively interact or interfere with any medications, including antibiotics, ADHD medication, birth control, acne medications, and allergy medications. Essentially, if you or a person you are tending to is taking medication of any kind, I urge you to do more extensive research and to discuss the use of herbal medicines with your healthcare professional(s). Do not stop or change prescription drug regimens without talking to your primary care provider or doctor.

Herbs and the Digestive System and the Adrenals

As the body grows during puberty, appetites run rampant, sugar is turned to as a source of energy, and hormones are flowing into every corner of the body. These elements can oftentimes contribute to an overworked and underappreciated digestive system. Proper absorption, elimination, and digestive health is important at this time. During puberty, our bodies are building their foundation and they need all of the support they can get. Some great herbs to turn to during this time include Tulsi, St. John's Wort, and a Tummy Healing tea blend.

Tulsi, also known as Holy Basil (*Ocimum tenuiflorum*) is a sweet, minty-tasting Ayurvedic herb which contains adaptogenic, blood sugar-stabilizing properties. Tulsi's nervous system regulating actions can help quell stress and anxiety related digestive upset. This plant is known for its spiritual properties which actively assists in breaking habits, possibly due to its ability to create a more peaceful environment for tackling such challenges. Combined with its blood sugar-balancing actions, it is a great option for those looking to quell an overdependence on sugar.

Suggested Use: As a tea or tincture.

If an overdependence on sugar is present, **St. John's Wort** (*Hypericum perforatum*) is another great plant to turn to. It is a powerful hepatic, which means that it tones, strengthens, and encourages the flow of bile in the liver. When large amounts of sugar, or processed foods have been consumed, St. John's Wort can aid the body in clearing the sluggishness from the system with more speed. Because of its power to clear the liver, do NOT take St. John's Wort if you are on ANY prescription medications. It is also known to increase photosensitivity, so do not take this herb and spend excessive amounts of time exposed to sunlight.

Suggested Use: As a tea or tincture.

If extensive damage has occurred to the digestive system through prescription medications such as antibiotics and ADHD medications or a diet heavy in fried foods, sugar, and processed foods, the following **Tummy Tea blend** is one I have used with many clients to promote healing and restore harmony in the gut microbiome, which is oftentimes destroyed or disturbed by the aforementioned things. This blend is meant to be used over a long period of time, ranging from one month to one year, daily, depending on how much healing is required in the digestive system. This is a general formula and may need to be adjusted according to your needs.

Tummy Tea Formula:

- *Calendula flower (Calendula officinalis)* is a plant that is a spectacular wound healer, especially in the digestive system. It's also chock-full of essential vitamins, such as A, B, D, and E. Its assistance to the lymph moves fluids and enhances elimination, which all point back to a well-rounded digestive system.
- *Chamomile flower (Matricaria recutita)* is flavorful, calming, and carminative. It is slightly bitter, which is a taste that promotes healthy bile release and thus, digestion.
- *Ginger root (Zingiber officinale)* is warming and dispersive. It stokes digestive fire through gingerol, a plant constituent that encourages healthy absorption and movement of food through the digestive system.
- *Turmeric root (Curcuma longa)* holds a golden color akin to the sacral chakra, of which the digestive system is a part of. Its antioxidant and anti-inflammatory properties are known to contribute to healthy digestion and assimilation of the nutrients in food. Curcumin, a plant compound in turmeric, stimulates bile production which can assist the body in digesting fats.
- *Rose petal (Rosa sp.)* is cooling, balancing, and calming to the digestive system. It is a harmonious addition to this blend which encourages regular bowel movements.
- *Peppermint (Mentha piperita)* is an antispasmodic herb enriched with the plant constituents menthol, which promotes the relief of gastrointestinal issues such as indigestion, bloating, cramping, and gas. It aids in normalizing digestive functions and makes a delicious accompaniment to this blend.
- *Rosemary (Salvia rosmarinus)* may be an ally to bloating, indigestion, gas, and stomach cramping. It is known to assist in the process of breaking down fats, which is something that can be impaired with digestive systems that are weakened.
- Optional but highly recommended addition: *Marshmallow root (Althaea officinalis)* offers mucilaginous, demulcent

properties to remedy damaged mucous membranes in the digestive system. It will soothe, repair, and bring moisture to inflamed tissues. If you find that this blend is too drying for you, Marshmallow root may be the plant you will want to add in to harmonize and balance this blend.

To make this Tummy Tea blend, simply place one part of each herb (with the exception of Marshmallow root—more on that below) in a bowl and blend together with clean hands or a spoon. Place two tablespoons of the formula in a french press or quart jar. Top with hot water and allow to steep, with a lid on, for 15 minutes. Strain and drink throughout the day. Any leftover tea may be kept in the fridge for 1 to 2 days. If you have not tried one of the herbs included, I recommend trying it individually as a cup of tea prior to using it in the blend.

NOTE: Marshmallow root should not be placed directly in the blend with the other herbs. Its medicinal qualities are brought out through cold to room temperature water extractions and mostly destroyed with heat. Simply place one teaspoon of marshmallow root to 8 oz of room temperature water and allow to steep for up to 8 hours. Strain and combine with cooled down healing Tummy Tea. Marshmallow root may also block the absorption of medications or supplements. It is recommended to take supplements 2 hours apart from when you use this herb.

Herbs for Your Skin and the Digestive System

Skin issues such as acne, eczema, and psoriasis are directly connected with the digestive and lymphatic systems in what researchers call the gut-skin axis.[101] Commonly, folks reach for topical treatments as the resolution for chronic skin issues. Topical treatments alone, from a holistic health perspective, fail to consider the internal landscape, which will bring us to the root cause of these skin imbalances. Our pathways of

101 S. Widhiati, D. Purnomosari,T. Wibawa., H. Soebono, "The Role of Gut Microbiome in Inflammatory Skin Disorders: A Systematic Review," *Dermatology Reports*, (2021), doi.org/10.4081/dr.2022.9188.

eliminating toxins and waste from the body include urine, sweat, feces, bile, saliva, tears, and our breath. When these are blocked, or not functioning properly, our bodies will express this disruption. For many people, especially during puberty, this happens through the skin.

Constipation, bloating, gas, diarrhea, nausea, and inability to sweat are other signs that the pathways of elimination are being disrupted. The following herbal suggestions may be applied here as well to provide support to the liver and digestive system.

Burdock root (*Arctium lappa*) also known as Gobo, is cooling, sweet, and moistening. It is rich in prebiotics, which are essential food sources for the healthy prebiotic bacteria that live in your gut. Its diuretic qualities assist in urination and sweating. Burdock stimulates lymph action that possibly leads to improved liver function. It is also known to be hepatoprotective, meaning that it prevents damage to the liver. Burdock has a true affinity for clearing and purifying the blood, which oftentimes can result in the clearing of skin issues.

Herbal medicines such as burdock are slow working medicines. To experience its effects, it is recommended to diligently drink daily infusions of burdock root for at least 2 weeks. As Burdock is a root, it must be decocted. Burdock is also a root that is eaten as a food and oftentimes found in health food or Asian grocery stores. Consider implementing it into your diet on days where you forget or do not want to make an infusion.

SAFETY NOTE: Burdock root should not be taken alongside blood thinners, diabetes medications, or other diuretics. As it moves fluids efficiently throughout and out of the body, be sure to drink plenty of water when using this plant.

Bitters are commonly an alcohol-based tincture prepared with a combination of bitter, aromatic, and carminative herbs. They often include plants such as chamomile, orange peel, dandelion root, ginger root, fennel, angelica root, gentian root, and burdock root. Using bitters prior to eating assists in the body preparing the gut for food via stimulating and releasing bile necessary for healthy digestion. Bitters are specifically recommended for instances when digestion is stagnant, when there is a lack of bitter elements in the diet, when strong cravings are present, or when frequent eating due to emotions occurs. While bitters are typically taken in tincture format, a bitter tea can be made as well if abstaining from alcohol. This medicine is most effective when taken 15 to 20 minutes prior to eating all meals.

Herbs for General Menstrual Support

Though they have been ascribed as a normal part of the menstruation process, intense pain, overwhelming bloating, and drastic mood changes—alongside other symptoms associated with the time before or during bleeding—are not actually standard for this phase. Our energy naturally wanes during menstruation, as this is the time in our cycle to encourage rest and slow movement. But pain? Heavy bleeding? Extremely long or short cycles? Not so much. These symptoms are signs that a root cause and imbalance needs to be addressed.

The next chapter dives more deeply into ways to support and nourish irregular menstruation conditions. The following touches on a few basic supportive plants for menstruation in general.

Raspberry leaf (*Rubus idaeus*) is an herb best used as a tonic, but which can also be used acutely for support during painful menstruation. It is rich in antioxidants such as polyphenols and anthocyanins, whose anti-inflammatory effects can help alleviate cramps. Raspberry leaf is also rich in vitamins and minerals, such as iron, magnesium, zinc, calcium, and vitamins C and E, which are nutrients needed to restore the body during and after bleeding.

This herb is known to tone and strengthen the uterine muscles when used over time, which encourages the healthy flow of blood and will thus prevent cramping. Consider taking daily raspberry leaf infusions for the week prior to menstruation, as well as during menstruation.

When acute pain from menstruation occurs, the first herb I turn to is **cramp bark** (*Viburnum opulus*). Its bark contains methyl salicylate, a plant compound which brings relief to minor aches, pains, and muscle cramps. As it relaxes tense uterine muscles, blood flows more readily, easing pain. A tincture or decoction of this herb is the best way to work with this plant in this situation.

Vitex (*Vitex agnus-castus*), also called chasteberry or chaste tree, is an herb many hear of when researching herbs to support the female reproductive system. It is painted as the cure-all for hormone imbalances and fertility issues, much like turmeric or curcumin is looked at for inflammation. However: there is no such thing as a cure-all. As discussed in the review of herbal energetics, every individual has varying needs and things to consider when applying plants to their bodies. If an herb sounds like your savior, I beg you to adjust your mindset to avoid being disappointed in the long-run. There are root causes of our symptoms at play. Consider your lifestyle habits first. Herbs second.

With that in mind, vitex contains wonderful properties with an affinity for the womb. This spicy, warming herb is known to decrease breast pain associated with PMS, likely due to its ability to raise progesterone levels and lower prolactin levels. For those in puberty who are coming off of birth control pills and do not experience the return of their menses, this may be a viable option for recalibration of hormones. However, this plant will not work miracles if other lifestyle factors do not shift, such as diet and stress load. Vitex must be used consistently on a short-term basis to experience these shifts, as, like many herbs, it is slow acting.

Again, this plant will not fix long-term chronic issues and is not specifically recommended to all people experiencing hormonal imbalances. Vitex should not be used for those who are anemic, chronically fatigued, or depressed/have a history of depression (as it can cause symptoms to worsen). Additionally, if you are low in B vitamins, magnesium, and Omega-3s, I do not recommend experimenting with vitex.

For those choosing to implement vitex in a protocol, it is recommended to start with a low dose: 10 drops in water, 2 to 3 times a day, for up to 6 months. If you are unsure about how to proceed with this herb, consider consulting a clinical herbalist or naturopath who is well-versed in herbalism and vitex.

Herbs for PMS and Emotional Support

Turbulent times may arise during puberty, whether it's in the form of general emotional distress, PMS, or both. PMS symptoms, which we will go into more deeply in the next chapter, includes mood swings, breast tenderness, depression, cravings, fatigue, and irritability. When PMS is chronically experienced, it is essential to start with addressing lifestyle factors such as diet, movement/exercise, stressors, and the general state of the mental space.

The herbs discussed in this section are known to assist on a spiritual and emotional level, which can create a good foundation for dealing with PMS symptoms. My favorite and most recommended herbs for emotional support include linden, hawthorne, and rose.

Linden (*Tilia*) is a cooling, relaxing, and uplifting nourishing herb which is tenderly referred to as "a hug in a mug." The leaves and flowers have gentle nervine qualities which are known to ease the mind, reduce anxiety, and calm nervousness. If nervous, tense headaches routinely occur, consider employing a cup of linden tea. It is floral, slightly sweet, and embodies a tranquil energy, especially when lightly sweetened with honey. If deep, chronic stress is present, this herb may be successfully used as a tonic in the form of daily infusions. When brewed in room temperature water, its mucilaginous properties shine, offering a cooling effect to any fiery feelings that may be occurring.

Hawthorn (*Crataegus spp.*) is a tree whose leaves, flowers, and berries are used in herbal medicine to tend to an over-anxious, depressed, worried, or disheartened state. Its medicine has been used for centuries as an energetically and physically protective tonic for the heart space. Hawthorn trees bear sharp, woody thorns which can be found on its trunk and stems. In witchcraft, the magickal, protective properties of this tree have been seen to offer guidance in stepping into new paths and to welcome new beginnings. Its berries are packed full of antioxidants, which clear out free radicals and directly repair the cardiovascular system. Additionally, this herb contains flavonoids, which have appeared to be protective to heart tissue and arterial walls.[102] Consider using this plant meditatively, as a tea, or tincture.

It is no secret that **rose** (*Rosa sp.*) is often associated with a heart heavy with emotions and stress. Here, we use the petals, which are aromatically rich, cooling, and astringent. Its cooling actions clear heat, which is often associated with anger and resentment. Rose is protective in spiritual and emotional ways, allowing the heart to soften and remain open while also protected and boundaried. In this situation, rose hydrosol is recommended topically as an aromatic and facial mist, daily. Rose tea or tincture may also be applicable and effective when a person is feeling closed, shameful of their development or actions, or if they are depressed. Note that rose is drying when

---

102 "Roles and Mechanisms of Hawthorn and Its Extracts on Atherosclerosis: A Review," *Frontiers in Pharmacology*, (2017), ncbi.nlm.nih.gov/pmc/articles/PMC7047282/.

taken internally over a period of time. To balance this, consider pairing with a moistening plant such as linden or violet leaf or flower. Additionally, rose pairs harmoniously for emotional support with tulsi, chamomile, and linden.

Herbs for Stress

As the body undergoes changes, it experiences a medley of stressors: From hormones to mental turmoil to fear to overexcitement to an abundance of strong emotions. These stressors send off a cascade of stress responses into the body. On top of this, the overprescribing of medications afflicts the majority of teenagers with rampant mineral and vitamin deficiencies. Adrenal burnout is likely to occur as they are glands that sit on top of the kidneys, which produce hormones to manage the stress response.

Plant medicines that may help during this time include lemon balm, milky oats, and nettle leaf.

Lemon balm (*Melissa officinalis*) is a bright nervine known to soothe and nurture overactive emotional states that may be ever-present for those in puberty. It is aromatically uplifting, calming, and elevating herb with an affinity for the nervous system and digestive system, which can be impacted with chronic stress. This herb contains rosmarinic acid, which is an anti-inflammatory and antioxidant that may assist in curbing inflammation caused by chronic stress. Its gentle nervine qualities supports quality sleep and encourages ease and peace for a tense constitution. Stress weakens the immune system, putting it at risk for cold sores to creep in. Lemon balm's antiviral applications, specifically in HSV, the virus that causes cold sores, blocks receptors on skin cells that allow the herpes virus to spread. Consider using lemon balm as a tincture, tea, or glycerite.

Milky oats (*Avena sativa*) is a tonic used to bring tremendous healing and nourishment to frazzled nervous systems. Milky oats are the fresh tops of oats, harvested when they are at the stage where they release a white, milky sap that is full of nutrients. This sap contains bioactive compounds restorative to the nervous system which coats frazzled, fatigued, and overworked nerves. As a whole, it supports our endocrine system by assisting in regulating hormones and bringing demulcent qualities to our glands. This plant is best used as a tincture, which is typically made when the oat tops are at the height of their milky stage, fastening the properties in the extraction. However, daily herbal infusions made with the dried plant are also helpful when used as a tonic over a long period of time.

Nettle leaf (*Urtica dioica*) brings restorative, nutrient dense qualities which are needed when the adrenals are overworked. The seat of the adrenals, the kidneys, are supported by nettle through its diuretic, cleansing qualities which are clearing and strengthening. Spiritually, this cleansing effect is considered to be a supportive place where emotions feel safe to be felt. Nettle leaf is a powerhouse of nutrition. It contains iron, magnesium, potassium, chlorophyll, Vitamins A, C, E, F, K, and P, and zinc. It is incredibly restorative to a system ladened with the effects of chronic stress. If a person has had a diet that includes excessive processed foods, or if a person took years of medications or antibiotics, this may be a plant that will highly benefit their bodies. Nettle blends well with milky oats in daily infusions, which may be applicable as a tonic.

Herbs for the Quest to Rest

During puberty, teenagers should be ideally sleeping between 10 to 12 hours a night. While asleep, these bodies are busy building adult systems, bones, and brains, as well as clearing toxic wastes from the brain.[103] When sleep is disrupted, this process is disrupted, which can lead to chronic health issues.

---

103 "Deep Sleep Takes Out the Trash," *ScienceDaily*, January 21, 2021, sciencedaily. com/releases/2021/01/210120151044.htm.

In the quest for rest, we want to aim to answer these questions with a yes or a change in lifestyle:

- Is the diet nourishing and appropriate for the individual?
- Are activating foods being left out of the diet?
- Is adequate movement/exercise happening on a daily basis?
- Are stressors being mitigated where appropriate and possible?
- Are creative pursuits being pursued and made a priority?

While herbs may be applied to support a person having difficulty with sleep, whether or not they can say yes to all of the above questions, these factors will likely impact how effectively those herbs work. Herbs can work to support curbing sleep/resting issues when there is an emotional or mental topic that is heavily present. Chamomile, skullcap, and ashwagandha are supportive herbs that nourish the nervous system and promote the deep relaxation needed for proper sleep.

Chamomile (*Matricaria chamomilla*) is a relaxing nervine with antispasmodic qualities. If restless tension, anxiety, and racing thoughts are an issue, chamomile medicine may be an effective application. Its antispasmodic qualities may be of benefit to those who experience a lack of sleep due to headaches or issues with digestion. It pairs well with tulsi, lemon balm, passionflower, mint, and skullcap in the form of a bedtime tea. Additionally, for those who may be adverse to tea, its relaxing effects may also be experienced through bathing with a strong infusion of the tea or used as a tincture.

Skullcap (*Scutelleria spp.*), a nervine from the mint family, has been historically used by Native Americans. This herb is energetically drying and cooling, relaxing the nervous system while rebuilding nerve structures. It helps the body release tense and stressful energy in a more sustainable and healthy way. For those who experience strong emotions, fear, irritability, and utter exhaustion, skullcap may be a great ally. While this plant beholds powerful qualities, it is gentle enough for overall relaxation that it may also be taken during the day. It pairs well with mint, lemon balm, and rose.

Ashwagandha (*Withania somnifera*) is an adaptogenic herb used in Ayurvedic medicine for centuries and has been recently embraced by western herbalism. Ashwagandha's adaptogenic properties help the body adapt to stress more effectively. It may also enhance sleep quality as it contains triethylene glycol, which is highly beneficial to restorative sleep. These qualities assist the body in restoring a healthy sleep/wake cycle.

SAFETY NOTES: Those with a baseline energy level of fatigue may find that this plant exasperates this state. It is also contraindicated for those with diabetes, an intolerance to nightshade plants, low/high blood pressure, and stomach ulcers. It may also not be the right fit for those with autoimmune or thyroid disorders as it may be too stimulating.

Mother: Applicable Herbs during Pregnancy and Postpartum

Traditionally, plants have been used for all of human existence by birth workers and women to greatly support and nourish a pregnant and breastfeeding body. As you will see, there are many overlapping herbs for both when the baby and body are developing during pregnancy and when the baby has been born. These nourishing plants support the development of babies and contain nutrients, minerals, and herbal actions that are much needed for the pregnant mother, as well as during breastfeeding.

It is important to consider what plants you are using during these times, especially during the first and second trimesters. While you may have herbs on hand which may initially sound supportive to symptoms being experienced, they may actually be detrimental and contraindicated in pregnancy. To prevent this, it is vitally important to do thorough research or work with an herbalist or healthcare provider, such as a midwife or clinical herbalist, to determine if an herb is right for you and your pregnancy or postpartum journey. While the plants that will be discussed in this section of the book are historically gentle, safe, and effective, it is essential that they are used and applied with mindfulness, with deep consideration, and in a safe way.

Herbs and Morning Sickness

In the first trimester, morning sickness, nausea, and difficulty with digestion are the most common stressors in pregnancy. These symptoms are exhausting and depleting, affecting not only the nervous systems, but the entire body. Frequent vomiting makes it difficult to maintain adequate nutrition.

Herbs such as ginger root and peach leaf may be of assistance here. Clinical trials have shown the efficacy of ginger root as an application to those experiencing morning sickness.[104]

Gingerol, the active compound in **ginger root** (*Zingiber officinale*), works with the digestive system to relieve nausea, bloating, vomiting and gastric distress. Ginger's energetics are warming, which may make it an unwise choice for those with a warm constitution or when hyperemesis[105] is present, which indicates that the tissue states are hot. In the case of morning sickness symptoms, its recommended use is through fresh ginger root as a decoction, or in powdered form as a tea. When the liquid has cooled, consider adding a touch of honey and sea salt to assist in replenishing and rehydrating the system. For those on the go, think about grabbing a ginger infused tincture, honey, or pastille.

Peach (*Prunus persica*) holds medicinal qualities that may be exceptionally applied to those who are pregnant. Its fruit,

---

104 "The Effectiveness of Ginger in the Prevention of Nausea and Vomiting during Pregnancy and Chemotherapy," *Integrative Medicine Insights*, (2016), ncbi.nlm.nih.gov/pmc/articles/PMC4818021/.
105 Hyperemesis is prolonged or severe vomiting.

leaf, seed, and bark are used as a cooling, demulcent nervine, which is great for those who are looking for a more cooling alternative to ginger. These qualities are brought out most vividly through a cold infusion of the leaves, and may provide instant relief to those experiencing vomiting, nausea, and anxiety related digestive issues. Peach medicine is known to be an herbal ally for those experiencing fatigue due to exhaustion from morning sickness, worry about the pregnancy, or general stress. In addition to these qualities, it is known to tone the uterine muscles, indicating that it pairs well with red raspberry leaf, which is typically used in the third trimester. As peach leaf may not be as readily available, ingesting it as a tincture in water may be more accessible.

Herbs and Nourishment during Pregnancy

Proper nourishment is crucial for the vitality of both the baby and the pregnant person and relies heavily on nutrition before, during, and after pregnancy. While the fetus undergoes key developmental stages, the pregnant body also grows and is in need of adequate nutritional support to stay healthy during and after birth. While foods consumed during this time should be focused on, herbs can come in to assist and supplement minerals and vitamins that we may be lacking. Three herbs known to be greatly supportive during pregnancy are nettle leaf, marshmallow root and rose hips.

If it has not already been made clear throughout this book, **nettle leaf** (*Urtica dioica*) is useful for all people in all walks of life. But, when it comes to pregnancy, this herb is used time and time again. And with good reason. Nettle is mineral and nutrient rich, surpassing the volume to nutrition ratios of spinach and many cultivated dark leafy greens. As a tonic, nettle leaf infusions may assist in the restorative process for hair loss that occurs during or after pregnancy due to mineral deficiencies. It is commonly referred to as "Mother Nature's breast milk," as it provides nutrition needed for breastfeeding and is considered a galactagogue, which is an herb that increases or maintains breastmilk production. Its diuretic qualities are known to be an effective remedy for edema and leg swelling that tends to occur during the second and third trimester.

As discussed previously, if nettle is too drying, consider combining it with a cold infusion of marshmallow root. Marshmallow root's wonderful cooling and moistening properties may be helpful if heartburn or indigestion is present as it assists in healing mucous membranes and encouraging healthy elimination, which can sometimes be halted by first trimester constipation.

Rose hips (*Rosa spp.*) are rich in bioavailable Vitamin C—essential for the baby's physical development, enhancing nutrient absorption—and act as an antioxidant to protect cells from inflammation. This plant medicine also contains magnesium, calcium, and healthy fatty acids. Like rose petals, rose hips assist in circulation of blood throughout the body and act as a mild diuretic, benefiting those experiencing edema or looking to strengthen their immune system. Rose hips should always be used in their whole form as a decoction and not ingested as an essential oil.

SAFETY NOTE: It is recommended by some that rose hips should not be used within the first month of pregnancy.

Herbs and Anxiety/Stress during Pregnancy

Pregnancy is often considered a time for sacred growth. However, the expectation that one must glow with happiness throughout the entire nine months doesn't reflect the reality of many. Instead, this time may include periods marked by distress, anxiety, and increased stress for a variety of reasons.

It is essential to adopt healthy habits and tools to cope with these intense feelings during and after pregnancy. To bring balance to the nervous system, it is essential to focus on finding aligned tools and practices that offer peace and clarity. Consider visiting Chapter 8 on holistic practices for the menstrual cycle. Practices such as body scanning, breast massage, journaling, meditative walking, spending time in nature, and gentle breathwork may be helpful here. In tandem with these practices, you may implement herbal medicine to support the nervous system. Nervines generally safe during pregnancy include lemon balm and chamomile.

Lemon balm (*Melissa officinalis*) aromatics alone are mood boosting, uplifting, comforting and soothing. An infused oil, made with fresh lemon balm leaves, will allow you to experience its therapeutic aromatherapy and may be used in the same fashion as a lotion, all over the body. When used internally, lemon balm is known for its gentle nervine effects, relieving stress and anxiety while calming frazzled nerves. This herb is known to be an effective remedy against insomnia as it offers a calm energy for an overactive mind. For those who experience herpes simplex virus, this herb may be a wise choice in preventing the onset of an outbreak, which has a tendency to occur during pregnancy. Lemon balm combines well with nettle and chamomile as a tea and is gentle enough to imbibe throughout the day without affecting most people's alertness.

Chamomile flowers (*Matricaria chamomilla*) are another exceptional, gentle nervine which tends to those experiencing tension and/or repetitive thoughts. When combined with nettle leaf, it is truly nourishing and restorative, helping resolve or mitigate depletion and exhaustion. For those experiencing chronic anxiety, I recommend taking a bath with a strong infusion of its blossoms. Do note that some people have allergies to chamomile, as it is in the Asteraceae family. As such, it should be used with caution to those who have not used it previously.

Red Raspberry Leaf and the Third Trimester

Red raspberry leaf (*Rubus idaeus*) is widely known to be the star herbal ally of the third trimester of pregnancy, as it has been historically used to prepare the body for delivery of a baby. It is thought that its nutrient-dense composition strengthens and tones the uterine muscles which allow for a smoother and faster delivery with minimal bleeding. In preparation for labor, we want to ensure adequate, essential nourishment is prioritized so the body processes and anatomy—uterine muscles included—are regulated and functioning in a healthy way.

Studies have shown that those who drank infusions of red raspberry leaf may also be less likely to experience preterm labor, need a C-section, or need forceps or a vacuum during birth.[106] However, while this plant is mostly documented to be a supportive herb, some studies have shown that it is also known to stimulate uterine muscle contractions, which is why it may need to be avoided for those at risk for early labor. It is also why raspberry leaf is generally not recommended during the first trimester.

Herbs for Postpartum Care

After birth, the body is undergoing a vast amount of changes in a short period of time: Breast milk may be coming in. The uterus is shrinking. Lochia, the bloody, vaginal discharge that occurs after birth, arrives. The perineum may be torn or extremely stretched and sore. And, deep exhaustion from labor is likely present. Receiving tender care, support, and nourishment are instrumental during this time to revitalize the postpartum body and to prepare oneself to tend to a new life.

Herbal baths for those who have given birth are not only calming to the nervous system, but directly healing to the areas which experienced trauma. These tender tissues necessitate

106 "Raspberry Leaf (Rubus idaeus) Use in Pregnancy: A Prospective Observational Study," *BMC Complementary Medicine and Therapies*, 2024.

gentle care. I suggest being mindful of avoiding products which contain essential oils, as they may further inflame and irritate tissue states. The following bath recipes can be mixed in advance and make an excellent gift for expecting parents. For those who experienced a C-section, these may be used as a relaxing foot bath.

Relax and Soothe Postpartum Bath

This blend is aromatically calming while offering skin healing and mending properties. Boil 2 quarts of water in a medium-sized pot. Turn off heat and add in 1 to 3 tablespoons of rose, yarrow, lavender, and chamomile followed by 2 cups of epsom or magnesium salts. Place the lid atop the pot and allow it to steep for 20 to 30 minutes. As it steeps, pour a warm bath. Strain the herbs from the water and pour tea directly into the bathtub, soaking for at least 20 minutes.

Deep Healing Postpartum Bath

This deep healing blend brings a medley of herbs known to promote wound healing and repair to bruised tissues. Boil 2 quarts of water in a medium sized pot. Turn off heat and add in 1 to 3 tablespoons of calendula, yarrow, plantain, and witch hazel followed by 2 cups of epsom or magnesium salts. Place the lid atop the pot and allow it to steep for 20 to 30 minutes. As it steeps, pour a bath. Strain and pour tea directly into the bathtub, soaking for at least 20 minutes. The use of magnesium salts further assists in promoting wound healing, reduction of inflammation, pain, and offers general relaxation of muscles and mind.

Heavenly Bum Spray

Additional healing may be brought in through Herbal Perineal Sprays, which can be applied to soothe the inflamed tissues of the perineum. The following is a recipe I make for expecting clients, friends, and family. If an allergy to any of these herbs is present, omit it and add in an additional part of floral hydrosol of choice in the ingredients list.

- 1 part Rose Hydrosol
- 1 part Witch Hazel Extract
- 1 part Lavender Hydrosol
- A dollop of cosmetic grade Glycerin
- A dollop of Vitamin E oil

Combine in a small bowl and whisk until fully combined. Pour into a spray bottle and label. Keep cold in the refrigerator for up to 6 months.

Herbs and C-Section

Those who experience a C-section birth experience postpartum recovery differently, as they are recovering from a surgery which may have been elective, planned, or emergency in nature. C-section births take an average of 6 to 8 weeks to heal tissues compared to vaginal births, which take an average of 2 to 6 weeks. As major surgery has taken place, it is important to seek rest, nourishment from warming slow-cooked foods, and ample hydration. Here we can implement herbs such as ginger root and turmeric to promote circulation and for their wound healing properties.

Digestion may be negatively impacted as c-section surgery involves the abdomen area. To alleviate some of the uncomfortable symptoms that arise with this, **ginger root** (*Zingiber officinale*) may be a good option for its effects on the digestive system and overall circulatory support. Ginger's anti-inflammatory and warming properties work to move stagnant energy and amplify the digestive fire needed to prevent constipation or calm a spastic belly.

Topically, **turmeric** (*Curcuma longa*) has been shown in studies to promote the healing of c-section wounds.[107] It has also been used in ayurvedic medicine internally in conjunction with topical applications to bring healing to the wound site.

Golden milk—an ancient ayurvedic recipe that contains ginger, turmeric, and cinnamon (another herb which promotes healing with its circulatory stimulating energetics)—is an elixir which can be employed as a tonic post C-section.

Golden Milk Recipe
- 8 oz. of raw cow's, coconut, almond, or hemp milk
- 1 teaspoon turmeric
- A pinch of black pepper
- .5 teaspoon Ceylon cinnamon
- .25 teaspoon ginger
- A pinch of cardamom (optional)
- A small squeeze of honey (optional)

Pour choice of milk in a small saucepan over medium heat. As the temperature slowly rises, whisk in herbs, continuing to stir as liquid warms. When almost simmered, remove from heat and allow to steep for 8 minutes. Using a fine-mesh strainer, pour in mug of choice. When lightly cooled, add honey if desired.

Herbs and Breastfeeding
Using herbal medicine to support and encourage breast milk supply is not one-size-fits-all. Locating the root cause as to why breast milk may be delayed, drying up, not present at all, or supplied in an overabundance can sometimes be difficult to pinpoint. Because of this, I will discuss both herbs that are ultimately holistically nutritive and supportive, nettle leaf and

---

107 G. Mahmudi, M. Nikpour, M. Azadbackt, R. Zanjani, M. A. Jahani, A. Aghamohammadi, and Y. Jannati, "The Impact of Turmeric Cream on Healing of Cesarean Scar," *West Indian Medical Journal*, July 7, 2015, doi.org/10.7727/wimj.2014.196.

marshmallow root, as well as two commonly recommended plants to support breastfeeding, vitex and fennel seed.

As always: before herbs, address lifestyle. It is very important to focus on proper hydration and adequate nourishing foods to promote steady production of milk.

Nettle leaf (*Urtica dioica*) has a profound nutritional prowess during breastfeeding and is known for optimizing milk production and restoring the body with nutrients and minerals lost through the process of breastfeeding. Using nettle as a food or through infusions are generally very useful, safe, and supportive.

Marshmallow root (*Althaea officinalis*) is also a star player in soothing the breasts during this high-impact time. If breasts are swollen, tender, or raw, a cold infusion of this herb may be prepared for topical and internal use. For topical use, strain and pour tea in a bowl that is wide and shallow enough to soak breasts in, or soak a soft wash cloth in the tea and place directly on the breasts. This will soothe and cool the inflamed skin, recovering the tissues from breastfeeding. Internally, marshmallow's moistening properties promote hydration and coat the mucous membranes from the mouth to the anus, protecting tissues, keeping tissues hydrated and supple, and encouraging healthy digestion.

As the postpartum body experiences its many hormonal shifts, low doses of **vitex** (*Vitex agnus-castus*) on a short-term basis may assist in re-regulating hormones. Vitex may be used to increase breast milk production; however, it's also known to decrease breast milk production via inhibiting prolactin production. This varies from person to person and is dependent on one's constitution and the root cause behind a lack or surplus of breast milk. This herb demonstrates why choosing herbs to support breastfeeding can be tricky without clinical experience or the help of a healthcare provider. SAFETY NOTE: As always, it is important to seek the recommendations of your herbalist, midwife, or healthcare prior to using vitex. For more details, see "Herbs for General Menstrual Support."

Fennel seed (*Foeniculum vulgare*) is an herb commonly found and recommended in breast milk tea blends as well as in lactation cookies. This herb is rejuvenating, antispasmodic, and carminative, and through these actions, reduces inflammation in the mucous membranes of the digestive system. It stokes digestive fire, allowing for better absorption of foods and more timely elimination. These attributes are often favored for breastfeeding babies that experience colic and digestive upset. Fennel seed is also known to increase breast milk supply fat content, which ultimately can assist in infant weight gain. Like vitex, fennel can increase or decrease milk supply, depending on constitution, tissue state, and the body's needs, as it is a mild diuretic. Because of this quality, it may be of assistance to those who are experiencing after birth swelling/edema. I do not recommend using fennel seed oil, but the whole seed itself in the form of a decoction. Fennel may pair well with fenugreek, which is also traditionally used in breast milk teas and lactation cookies.

Herbs known to decrease breast milk supply include sage, oregano, peppermint, thyme, and yarrow.

Herbs and Postpartum Brain Fog

Brain fog is a common experience for those who have just given birth. The body is undergoing changes, deep healing, and, well, there is a new baby to take care of at all hours of the day.

A combination of rest, adequate nourishment and hydration, and herbal medicine will assist in mitigating the effects of brain fog. Daily infusions of both **milky oats** (*Avena sativa*) and **nettle leaf** (*Urtica dioica*) offer nutritive qualities and nervous system nourishment. Milky oats have nootropic qualities that promote stability to the nervous system, which will aid in more restful, deep sleep. Nettle leaf synergizes the blend with its deeply nutritive qualities, acting to fill in any vitamins and minerals gaps.

For those who are not breastfeeding, internal use of **rosemary** (*Rosmarinus officinalis*) may be a welcomed herbal ally for brain fog. Rosemary is historically known for strengthening the memory and "waking up" the brain, which can be viscerally felt in its aromatics. Rosmarinic acid, a plant compound found in rosemary, moves stagnancy related to brain fog, tense anxiety, and exhaustion. Its antioxidant qualities eliminate free radicals, which cause damage to the body and are typically present with chronic fatigue. Use rosemary in food, as a tea, and as a syrup. For those who are breastfeeding, consider making a bath with rosemary, as its aromatic properties will also stimulate an alert mental state.

Rosemary Bath
- 3 to 4 tablespoons rosemary leaves
- 1 quart freshly boiled water
- .25 cup Epsom salts
- A french press or quart jar

Place rosemary leaves and epsom salts in a french press or quart jar and cover with hot water. Allow to steep for 30 to 45 minutes, covered. Strain and pour directly into warm bath. Soak inside of the bath for at least 20 minutes. Rinse off with a cold shower.

Postpartum Emotional Care

There is deep, incredible magick in having a new baby in one's life. There are also a deep amount of emotions that arise and which sometimes come all at once. Plant medicines have been used to support the healthy release and understanding of emotions for as long as plants and humans have existed. They are what our ancestors turned to in times where sometimes new, deep emotion was present. Two plants that may be highly beneficial for new mothers needing emotional support include motherwort and hawthorn.

Motherwort (*Leonurus cardiaca*) literally has the word mother in its name, and rightfully so, as it is a plant that is known to tend and nurture one's heart space. Motherwort's ability to hold space for grief, sorrow, and despair is far and wide. It is highly recommended to those experiencing PMDD or to those that may have experienced a pregnancy loss. In addition to its ability to tend to the emotional space, it is an emmenagogue, which stimulates and relaxes the uterus. Historically, it has been used to assist the body in the expulsion of lochia and the placenta. Motherwort pairs well with linden, hawthorn, and milky oats. As this herb is quite bitter, its medicinal qualities are best preserved and used as a tincture.

Hawthorn (*Crataegus spp.*) consistently shows up as a potent herbal ally when it comes to matters of the heart and mind-body connection. As mentioned in previous pages, its medicine benefits the cardiovascular system and is used as a plant that offers protection psychically and physically. The Hawthorn tree has been considered a source of enchanting protection in Celtic traditions. Its thick thorns, often used in protection spells and medicines, illustrate its protective nature. Hawthorn is warming and stimulating, making it useful for those who are feeling physically and emotionally cold, depressed, or despondent. It assists in moving emotion, softening edges that feel hard, and offering a sense of safety to those feeling unsure. SAFETY NOTE: There is little research on the safety of this herb with breastfeeding, so consult your healthcare provider prior to using or sharing with another.

Crone: Applicable Herbs for Menopause

As we discussed herbs to assist puberty, pregnancy, and postpartum, there are herbs that will support and nourish the body as it transitions from its reproductive years into menopause. I will not be making a distinction between herbs suggested during the separate phases of menopause as the symptoms experienced by individuals vary. This will be an overview of plants that will be supportive in every phase (unless otherwise noted).

Herbs for Deep Nourishment in Menopause

As estrogen declines and the overall hormonal landscape of a person in menopause greatly shifts, proper nourishment and support is needed to adjust for these changes. Without it, our bodies are more susceptible to damage from poor diet, alcohol consumption, and stress.

Nutritional needs for this time include ensuring adequate protein, calcium, magnesium, Vitamin D, and healthy fat sources are consumed. The amounts needed vary from person to person. The following are general suggestions and examples of what is generally recommended of each nutrient during or after menopause:

- 1,200 mg of Calcium
- 600 to 2,000 IU of Vitamin D3, through supplementation or direct sun exposure
- .7 to 1 gram of protein per pound of weight
- 300 to 320 mg of Magnesium
- 1 gram minimum of Omega-3s

It is preferable that these nutrients are obtained through diet or lifestyle. Taking too much of a supplement can have negative effects. In addition to supplements, there are herbs that are effective at both nourishing the body and supporting it in the other ways needed during menopause, which include red clover and nettle leaf.

Red clover (*Trifolium pratense*) is a nourishing herb historically used during menopause. Red Clover contains isoflavones, which in studies have shown great efficacy at reducing hot flashes and improving overall mood.[108] These compounds have the potential to have phytoestrogenic qualities, which means they have estrogenic or antiestrogenic effects. This is why red clover is typically contraindicated for those with hormonal disorders or estrogen-dependent breast cancer. Use red clover as a daily, overnight-steeped infusion or tincture.

As mentioned many times in this book, **nettle leaf** (*Urtica dioica*) is a source of essential vitamins and minerals that the body uses for optimal performance and function. That is why it absolutely has a place in nourishing the body during menopause. While it replenishes the body with great sources of nutrients, it may also support kidney function and health and is a key ally for UTIs. Nettle leaf may assist with those experiencing hair loss during menopause, specifically to those who are chronically depleted of essential nutrients. As suggested earlier, daily overnight infusions are the recommended way to consume nettle leaf. However, freeze dried nettle pills may be effective as well.

Herbs and Overall Dryness

Estrogen stimulates the body's oil and collagen production. When it declines, so does the oil and collagen content of one's skin. Because of this, the body is more susceptible to dryness.

Collagen is the most abundant protein in the body. It turns into connective tissue which connects all tissues. It strengthens skin and promotes flexibility in joints and muscles. It is what keeps our skin, bones, and joints supple, healthy, and lubricated. When collagen is lacking, it is essential to supplement collagen or collagen supportive herbs through one's diet. Herbs that may aid overall dryness include horsetail, marshmallow root, and CBD.

---

108 "Evaluation of Clinical Meaningfulness of Red Clover (Trifolium pratense L.) Extract to Relieve Hot Flushes and Menopausal Symptoms in Peri- and Post-Menopausal Women: A Systematic Review and Meta-Analysis of Randomized Controlled Trials." Nutrients, (2021), ncbi.nlm.nih.gov/pmc/articles/PMC8069620/.

Horsetail (*Equisetum arvense*) is a plant known for its high silica content, mineral-rich composition, and ability to strengthen bones. It contains calcium, potassium, magnesium, iron, and fatty acids, all of which are extremely important nutrients the body needs during the transition into menopause. Its silica-rich properties are known to maintain the health of bones and teeth, nourish connective tissue, and may even nourish arthritis through its ability to strengthen and improve elasticity of joints. Horsetail may be used as a tea, in powder form, as a tincture, or in capsules.

Marshmallow root (*Althaea officinalis*) is cooling, moistening, sweet, and relaxing—all greatly welcomed qualities when body systems are exasperated with heat. Marshmallow acts effectively with the reproductive and gastrointestinal systems, cooling inflamed tissues and blanketing dry tissues with its mucilaginous qualities. Cold water marshmallow infusions are beneficial in promoting rehydration of skin and cells. The powder may be combined with water and turned into a paste, which may be applied topically. A washcloth soaked in a cold infusion and placed directly on the vulva is another way to bring relief to this area. Marshmallow may also be effectively employed as a daily infusion to prevent or lessen the frequency of hot flash spells. Consider pairing it with linden, which is also a cooling, nervous system balancing plant.

CBD, the non-psychoactive form of cannabis, when extracted into an oil, may be used as a suppository or directly applied to the vagina and vulva to support healthy lubrication to ease vaginal dryness. CBD has been noted to ease vaginal pain, ease penetration, and may heighten arousal for those having issues with libido. It is used both as a sexual lubricant and alone to relieve itchiness, dryness, and aggravation that is sometimes brought forth through menopause.

Herbs and Kidney Support

Menopause and kidney health are inextricably linked. Studies have shown that the health of kidney function becomes impaired as the hormonal cascade in the body shifts.[109] As estrogen levels decrease, the risk of kidney disease increases,[110] and those with pre-existing kidney disease may also be at risk for early menopause.[111] Notably, a 2008 study showed that long-term use of oral estrogen replacement therapy may negatively impact renal function.[112]

So, what can folks do to ease the effects these hormonal changes have on kidney health? The same thing that has been recommended time and time again in this book: Be intentional about lifestyle choices. Eat a well-balanced diet with a focus on fresh foods. Make it a priority to get in adequate movement and exercise each day. Keep a mindful eye on blood sugar and drink plenty of water. In addition to these lifestyle factors, nettle root may be supportive to kidney function.

While we have explored nettle leaf in length, its root contains very different medicinal properties. **Nettle root** (*Urtica dioica*) is known to be an effective remedy in pelvic stagnation and overall toning of the kidneys. Like its leaf, the root is a

109 Catherine Kim, Rajiv Saran, Michelle Hood, Carrie Karvonen-Gutierrez, Mia Q. Peng, John F. Randolph, and Siobán D. Harlow. "Changes in Kidney Function During the Menopausal Transition: The Study of Women's Health Across the Nation (SWAN) – Michigan Site," *Menopause 27*, no 9 (June 15, 2020): 1066–69. doi.org/10.1097/gme.0000000000001579.

110 "Chronic Kidney Disease and the Involvement of Estrogen Hormones in its Pathogenesis and Progression, (June 1, 2012), *PubMed,* pubmed.ncbi.nlm.nih.gov/23326957/.

111 D.Qian, Z. Wang, Z., Y. Cheng, R. Luo, S. Ge, and G. Xu, "Early Menopause May Associate with a Higher Risk of CKD and All-Cause Mortality in Postmenopausal Women: An Analysis of NHANES," 1999–2014. Frontiers in Medicine, 9, (2022), doi.org/10.3389/fmed.2022.823835.

112 Sofia B. Ahmed, Bruce F. Culleton, Marcello Tonelli, Scott W. Klarenbach, Jennifer M. MacRae, Jianguo Zhang, and Brenda R. Hemmelgarn, "Oral Estrogen Therapy in Postmenopausal Women Is Associated With Loss of Kidney Function." *Kidney International* 74, no 3 (August 1, 2008): 370–76, doi.org/10.1038/ki.2008.205.

mild diuretic and acts to assist the body in complete urination, which may become more difficult during and after menopause. The root is also known to relieve the feeling that one needs to constantly urinate. Additionally, nettle root keeps testosterone and estrogen active in the body for a longer length of time.

Decoction of the root, tincture, or capsules are appropriate here. If kidneys are already damaged or weakened, it is imperative that you seek the advice of a health care provider prior to taking this herb.

Herbs and Menopausal Heat

Hot flashes and night sweats are two symptoms that come up most when talking to friends, family, and clients who are experiencing menopause. Hot flashes occur as estrogen decreases. The lack of estrogen signals to the hypothalamus, which is the part of your brain that regulates body temperature, a message, "It's too hot in here." And as the hypothalamus's job is to regulate the body's temperature, it creates a cascade of processes to cool down the body, which includes hot flashes and night sweats.

While lifestyle changes can support the body in coping with this excessive heat, there are herbs that will directly support and nourish the body in this way as well. They include garden sage, motherwort, St. John's Wort, and peach leaf.

Garden sage (*Salvia officinalis*) is a mint family plant stimulating to the circulatory system and dispersive in nature. While sage is a warming plant, the aforementioned qualities work to bring the heat that is trapped in the core of the body to the surface.

Sage also contains phytoestrogens, which are thought to assist in decreasing hot flashes and improving sleep quality. Additionally, sage is known to support digestion, and act as on the mind for clarity and mood support. Use sage as a tea, tincture or culinary herb.

Motherwort (*Leonurus cardiaca*) is a cooling, bitter, relaxing nervine that is grounding and calming. When the body's systems are flooded with hormones, its bitter qualities assist the liver in processing them. This herb has a long history of use in menopause for hot flashes as well as relaxing the nervous system to achieve deep sleep. It is protective to a body and mind that is exhausted due to anxiety and worry. Use motherwort as a tincture, daily, before meals as a bitter, or in the evening, before bed, as a relaxant.

I've mentioned that **peach leaf** (*Prunus persica*) is a cooling, relaxing nervine. But, it's worth mentioning again while denoting its efficacy with heat during menopause. As eating a peach on a hot summer day feels cooling to both the mind and body, its extracted medicine offers the same energy. Its moistening properties are expressed in a cold tea of peach leaf, which are welcomed to tissues experiencing an intense flash of heat.

Experiencing intense, internal heat day in and day out is exhausting and aggravating and can lead to chronic tension. In this, peach medicine is deeply restorative to the nervous system, offering cooling relaxation to the person burnt out from menopausal symptoms.

Herbs for the Mind and Sleep

Menopause is a stressful time for some. Distressing symptoms may affect sleep. A lack of sleep directly impacts the mood. And, the mind may be worried, aggravated, or unsure. Whatever the case may be, there are herbs known to support these changes such as gotu kola and passionflower.

Gotu kola (*Centella asiatica*) has been used in many cultures to improve brain function. This herb contains blood purifying and circulatory qualities, which promote blood flow to the brain, and may stoke overall energy and mental clarity. Research shows that gotu kola increases and supports brain plasticity[113] and protects it from oxidative stress,[114] which supports concentration and memory. A study done in 2020 showed that the combination of gotu kola, goji berry, and xnidium fruit could improve memory and encourage the release of nerve growth factor, which is what helps grow and maintain neurons.[115] SAFETY NOTE: Those with impaired liver function, past or present, should seek medical advice prior to using gotu kola. Additionally, gotu kola should not be used prior to and after surgery nor alongside diuretics, vasodilators, hypoglycemic medications, or cholesterol-lowering agents.

If heart palpitations, chronic stress, tension, nervous anxiety, or insomnia are present, **passionflower** (*Passiflora incarnata*) may be indicated. Its energetics are cooling, drying, and bitter. When anxiety makes it difficult to sleep, passionflower's sedative nervine qualities work directly on the central nervous system to promote rest and calming of the mind. Its antispasmodic attributes are effective in its use for muscle spasms relating to stress.

Passionflower medicine may be used as a tea, tincture, or combined with other herbs in a relaxing, sleepy-time smoking blend.

SAFETY NOTE: As passionflower contains sedative and hypnotic effects, use caution when using this herb and operating a motor vehicle.

---

113 "Acute Enhancing Effect of a Standardized Extract of Centella asiatica (ECa 233) on Synaptic Plasticity: An Investigation via Hippocampal Long-Term Potentiation," *Pharmaceutical Biology*, 2021.

114 C. Chen, W. Tsai, C. Chen, and T. Pan, "Centella asiatica Extract Protects against Amyloid β1–40-induced Neurotoxicity in Neuronal Cells by Activating the Antioxidative Defense System," *Journal of Traditional and Complementary Medicine*, 6, 362–369, (2016), doi.org/10.1016/j.jtcme.2015.07.002.

115 J. G. Choi, Z. Khan, S. M. Hong, Y. C. Kim, M. S. Oh, and S. Y. Kim. "The Mixture of Gotu Kola, Cnidium Fruit, and Goji Berry Enhances Memory Functions by Inducing Nerve-Growth-Factor-Mediated Actions Both in Vitro and in Vivo," Nutrients, 12, 1372, (2020), doi.org/10.3390/nu12051372.

Sleepy Smoke Blend

- Passionflower
- Lemonbalm
- Peppermint
- Cornsilk
- Rose Petal

Take 1 tablespoon of each herb and place them in a small bowl. Combine with hands. I suggest doing this while in prayer or as you are in deep thought about the intention you would like to have while smoking these herbs. Prepare your vessel, whether that is a pipe or a smoking paper. Crumble the herbs you will use between your fingers or in a mortar and pestle. And enjoy. Store the remaining herb in a glass container with a label.

Chapter Ten: Herbalism & Other Holistic Therapies for Other Womb Experiences

*T*o have a womb is to experience a medley of unique situations, each requiring their own individual care. Painful periods may arise at the onset of bleeding. Endometriosis, ovarian cysts, PCOS, miscarriage, abortion, and stillbirth are all things commonly experienced by women and people with wombs today. And, they're often things we are left in the dark about—with few easy-to-use resources to guide us on how to heal our bodies and bring light to issues that can cause emotional, physical, and mental heaviness.

In this chapter, I will discuss herbs specific to common womb experiences, pregnancy losses / releases, and conclude with herbs that will be of great assistance across the board for emotional support. We will also explore holistic practices that are supportive in these various womb circumstances. I touch on this in the pages to come, but it is important to know that the herbs and practices I share are not solely for physical relief but are also for womb witchery in general, which extends a hand to spiritual and emotional work and healing. NOTE: There will be overlap from section to section as pregnancy loss as a whole involves healing the womb and recovering from blood loss and/ or surgery. In my opinion, it's information worth repeating. I highly suggest reading through every section, as each herb discussed can be used in a multitude of ways for the body, beyond the scope of alternate womb experiences and pregnancy loss. Please remember to consult a healthcare provider before using these herbs so that timing after procedures and dosing is tailored for you and your specific needs.

Lifestyle Considerations for Womb Experiences

While I tend to veer away from blanket statements about what is best for our individual healing process, there are factors to consider that can be applied to nearly every individual. As I've suggested (many) times throughout this book, lifestyle factors are essential to consider when we are dealing with imbalances and/or looking to live in a way that focuses on preventing imbalances. The following are a few of these key factors to consider.

Fresh, Whole Foods

What we put into our bodies is the fuel which will directly impact all of our systems. To be clear: This isn't about shaming. Or, telling you that you must have a "perfect" diet. But, reviewing what we've been eating and drinking will likely give insight into health matters and any dysregulation that may be present. If bloating, indigestion, or general discomfort occurs after meals, this may be a sign that something in your diet is not working for you and possibly causing systemic inflammation. As discussed throughout the book, aiming to eat mostly whole, non-heavily-processed foods; organic, pasture-raised meats; wild-caught, low mercury fish; and healthy Omega-3 rich fats and oils, as well as minimizing sugar, caffeine, and alcohol intake are things that are known to improve inflammatory responses, balance hormones, and regulate blood sugar. Some find that food prepping makes it easier to ensure they stay within, or near, this framework. Or, finding a handful of meals that can be made quickly and efficiently with fresh ingredients without sacrificing taste or satisfaction. See the appendix for suggestions on food blogs that may make meal time easier.

The way you eat your food matters. Meals and snacks eaten when rushed and unfocused can result in food that is not properly broken down through chewing and swallowing air while eating, which may provoke a stress response that causes the metabolism to slow down. This results in poorly digested food, preventing the body from efficiently assimilating. Food is best eaten in a slow, deliberate way. It will bring more presence to your life, your body, and the way you are reacting to certain foods when sitting down and taking adequate time to eat meals.

Regular Elimination

Eating fresh foods will assist the body in regular elimination, which is important when hormonal imbalances are present. When we are not pooping regularly, this waste sits in our bodies, reabsorbing the toxins and hormones our body is trying to send out from our systems. If you are not having one healthy poop a day, here are some things you may want to try:

- Drink 10 to 13 8 oz glasses of water, daily
- Consider how much fiber you are receiving in your diet. Aim for 25 to 30 grams of fiber, daily. Healthy sources of fiber include flaxseed, psyllium husk, beans, and many vegetables. Aim to receive your fiber mostly from whole food sources. However, do note that psyllium husk and flaxseed may be contraindicated if constipation is present. Start slowly with adding these foods.
- Feed and proliferate healthy gut bacteria with prebiotics and probiotics. Foods rich in prebiotics include leeks, burdock root, dandelion root, apples, artichokes, bananas, and oats. For probiotics, aim for at least one serving of fermented foods, a good probiotic pill, or 2 to 3 oz in fermented beverages, daily.
- Daily, cold infusions of marshmallow root. Place one teaspoon of herb to 8 oz of room-temperature water. Allow to infuse overnight. Strain and drink throughout the day. You may increase to 1 Tbsp to a french press or quart of room-temperature water.
- Reduce external stress that you can control at all costs. Consider adopting breathwork, yoga, stretching practice,

or whatever works best for you to support your nervous system.

- Supplement with magnesium, which pulls water to the bowels and assists in timely elimination. Daily recommended doses start around 300 to 400 mg.
- When waking up in the morning, perform a gentle stomach massage near your bowels, accompanied by drinking a whole glass of water with a pinch of salt. This is an ayurvedic practice known to stoke digestive fire and support morning elimination.
- Drink warm water with lemon, as it is known to assist in bowel movements.

Movement

Human bodies were made to move. Regularly. As many in western society have sedentary jobs or lifestyles, we must be more intentional about getting enough movement. The standard recommendation is 150 minutes of moderately difficult exercise a week. That's around one half-hour, five days a week, of activities such as dancing, bicycling, yard work, swimming, pilates, and weight lifting.

However, each body has varying needs, restraints, and abilities. What one person requires will be different than what the person next to them needs. I recommend creating a movement practice that is regular, above all. Find activities that you like. If you hate going to the gym, do not start by going to the gym. Go on a hike. A bike ride. Maybe pull weeds for a few hours a week. What is most important is moving our bodies regularly. The how is up to you to decide.

Reduce Exposure to Toxins

Plastic, fragrance, BPA-lined cans, hair and skin products, perfumes, household cleaners, processed foods, over-the-counter medications, and on and on are laden with insidious toxins which act as disruptors to our hormonal landscape and our immune, lymphatic, and nervous systems.

A few ways to avoid exposure to toxins include:

- Storing dry goods and spices in glass containers. Use leftover glass jars!
- Trying to buy hair and skin products which contain natural ingredients and minimal preservatives (Look to avoid sulfates, parabens, phthalates, and fragrance.)
- Drinking liquids out of glass bottles and cups instead of plastic
- Make your own household cleaners[116] (This is incredibly easy AND cheap.)
- Food prepping your kitchen essentials, such as non-dairy milks, yogurts, breads, baked goods, and granola
- Choosing menstrual products that are organic and bleach free

Herbs and Dysmenorrhea

There are a medley of disorders associated with painful periods, which we will cover in the following pages. However, for general dysmenorrhea, we look to herbal allies such as cramp bark, ginger root, and raspberry leaf.

Cramp bark (*Viburnum opulus*) has a historical use as a uterine antispasmodic, although it is also known to work for spasms in other parts of the body. Its name says it all; it is the bark for cramps. And it is effective at its job. In my clinical and personal experience, cramp bark effectively relaxes muscle tissues that are tense and tight due to menstruation and is also effective at calming ovulation cramping (also called mittelschmerz). Using this plant as a decoction or tincture 2 to

---

116 One of my favorite DIY books, *Make Your Place: Affordable, Sustainable Nesting Skills* by Raleigh Briggs is a great resource on making your own non-toxic, homemade cleaning products and beyond.

3 days prior to bleeding will render the best results, but will also show effective results during acute situations.

Ginger root's (*Zingiber officinale*) warming, spicy energetics and circulatory stimulating attributes are welcomed for bringing relief during painful periods. This plant has a way of moving blood with a stagnant, cold pattern, which is a common issue with chronic dysmenorrhea. Its anti-inflammatory properties assist in alleviating pain, especially when combined with turmeric or cramp bark as a decoction or tincture.

Raspberry leaf's (*Rubus idaeus*) astringent, toning functions on the uterine muscles come in as a key ally for dysmenorrhea. A phytochemical in raspberry leaf, phytosterol, is thought to tone the reproductive system and relax smooth muscle, which is important for a well flowing blood pattern in the uterus during menstruation. Consider using it as a tonic, especially the week before bleeding, in the form of an infusion. Pair it with nettle leaf for deeper nourishing qualities or linden for a more nervous system supportive approach.

Holistic remedies that may provide comfort for painful periods include:

- Using heating pads or hot water bottles to alleviate discomfort and promote the release of constriction
- Gentle yoga positions or stretches that encourage the hips, lower back, and thighs to open
- Warm baths with magnesium salts; relaxing herbs such as lavender, chamomile, and rose; and possibly ginger root decoctions. Note that ginger root baths can be extremely warming. Start slowly with bathing with this plant: place 2 cups of decoction in the bath, and increase from there.
- Gentle breathwork, such as square breathing or alternate nostril breathing exercises

Herbs and PMS

As PMS symptoms vary, their root causes vary as well. However, I often see in my clinical practice that supplementation of magnesium and Omega-3s can be incredibly helpful to the general population experiencing PMS and PMDD. A standard recommendation is 300 to 400 mg a day of magnesium glycinate or citrate and 1 to 2 grams of high-quality Omega-3/DHA/EPA. In addition to these, the body may be further supported with nervine and adaptogenic herbs such as tulsi, milky oats, and passionflower.

Tulsi's (*Ocimum tenuiflorum*) adaptogenic nervine qualities support and strengthen the nervous system. This herb hails from India, is a highly revered plant in Hindu cultures, and was eventually brought to Greek Orthodox traditions. This is a plant I use often, as its grounding, calming qualities are welcomed when chronic stress, anxiety, or fatigue are present. Its energy feels like a soothing shoulder rub after a long day. It is warming, cooling, and sweet. It makes a delicious tea, tincture, or elixir and may be used as a tonic. Consider combining it with milky oats, rose petals, or skullcap. Those who have hypoglycemia, take anticoagulation drugs, or are pregnant should talk to their health care provider before using Tulsi.

Milky oats (*Avena sativa*) have trophorestorative qualities with an affinity for the nervous system and are a key feature as to why this plant is beloved during PMS. Its milky sap brings reparative healing qualities to an overworked, fried, and frazzled nervous system. As discussed in previous pages, these benefits are created with long-term, tonic use. Its milky sap is best preserved in tincture form, but it is also effective as a nourishing infusion. Consider pairing it with nettle leaf for extra nourishment from minerals and vitamins.

Passionflower (*Passiflora incarnata*) is a plant whose medicine is grounding and calming, especially when the mind finds it hard to reach a restful state. Note that much of what we know about Passionflower is thanks to the Indigenous people who worked with it for centuries prior to the colonization of the U.S. and the enslaved black people who learned of its medicinal uses. Passionflower is also known for its anti-spasmodic qualities, which may come in handy for PMS symptoms where premenstrual cramping is present. In addition to these calming, pain-relieving qualities, it is also used as a means to quiet the mind for sleep when insomnia is present. Consider using this plant as a tea or tincture. It pairs well with tulsi, skullcap, rose, or lemon balm.

Holistic strategies for PMS include implementing daily breathwork, gentle yoga, and womb massage during the luteal phase. It may be wise to carve out alone time a few days before you start bleeding for self-reflection through journaling, time in nature, or spending time doing a low-stress hobby.

Herbs and Endometriosis

Herbs commonly used in conjunction with supportive lifestyle shifts for endometriosis include peony root, ashwagandha, rhodiola rosea, and cramp bark.

White Peony Root (*Paeonia lactiflora*) also called Bai Shao in Traditional Chinese Medicine has been used for centuries in TCM and more recently in western herbalism for hormonal imbalances, in both female and male reproductive systems. While it is most commonly thought of as a PCOS herb, it has been shown to be a highly effective tonic for many individuals with endometriosis. Its bitter, sour qualities denote its effectiveness in working with the liver and assisting in decreasing inflammation. Peony is noteworthy for endometriosis due to its documented ability to work as a smooth muscle relaxant thanks to paeoniflorin, a phytochemical in white peony with analgesic[117] and antispasmodic qualities. Often, it is recommended as a tonic to be used daily. Use as a decoction or tincture, depending on one's reaction to alcohol.

Ashwagandha (*Withania somnia*) is warming, bitter, and somewhat drying. It's been historically used and cultivated in India as an Ayruvedic beloved herb used as an endocrine and immune system tonic. It is known to balance the effects of stress[118] and lower cortisol levels,[119] which is thought to regulate and enhance reproductive function.[120] As ashwagandha beholds fat soluble compounds, it is essential to imbibe this plant with a fat, such as milk, ghee, or coconut oil, to render it effective. However, as Ashwagandha may further chill out individuals who are already fatigued and low on energy, rhodiola rosea may be used alongside it to balance the scales.

Rhodiola rosea is known for its cognitive effects, such as boosting attention span, reducing fatigue, and offering mental clarity. Like ashwagandha, its adaptogenic qualities bring balance to stressful states through combating excessive cortisol release.[121] Ashwagandha and rhodiola are a generally supportive blend that those with endometriosis may find helpful

117 "CP-25, a Compound Derived from Paeoniflorin: Research Advance on Its Pharmacological Actions and Mechanisms in the Treatment of Inflammation and Immune Diseases," *Acta Pharmalogica Sinica*, 2020.

118 "Ashwagandha: Is It Helpful for Stress, Anxiety, or Sleep?", Office of Dietary Supplements, (n.d.), ods.od.nih.gov/factsheets/Ashwagandha-HealthProfessional/.

119 J. Salve, S. Pate, K. Debnath, and D. Langade "Adaptogenic and Anxiolytic Effects of Ashwagandha Root Extract in Healthy Adults: A Double-Blind, Randomized, Placebo-Controlled Clinical Study," Cureus, (2019), doi.org/10.7759/cureus.6466.

120 M. Wiciński, A. Fajkiel-Madajczyk, Z. Kurant, D. Kurant, K. Gryczka, M. Falkowski, M. Wiśniewska, M. Słupski, J. Ohla, Z. Zabrzyński, (2023b), "Can Ashwagandha Benefit the Endocrine System?—A Review, *International Journal of Molecular Sciences*, 24, 16513. doi.org/10.3390/ijms242216513.

121 E. Olsson, B. Von Schéele, A. Panossian, "A Randomised, Double-Blind, Placebo-Controlled, Parallel-Group Study of the Standardised Extract SHR-5 of the Roots of Rhodiola roseain the Treatment of Subjects with Stress-Related Fatigue," Planta Medica, 75, 105–112, (2008),doi.org/10.1055/s-0028-1088346.

in balancing the stress experienced from chronic pain and the interference it has on daily life. Rhodiola may be used as a tea, tincture, or in capsule form.

Cramp bark (*Viburnum opulus*), as mentioned in the dysmenorrhea section, is a highly effective tool for the chronic pain that usually comes alongside endometriosis. It acts as a uterine decongestant to soothe endometriosis symptoms, such as pain prior to bleeding, bloating, and delayed menstruation. As tension headaches may be present with this condition, cramp bark may be an effective application, especially when combined with wood betony, tulsi, or linden in a tincture or tea.

Lifestyle changes that may be wise to implement for endometriosis include:

- Ensuring sufficient Omega-3s are being consumed, whether through regular consumption of wild-caught fish or supplementation
- Reducing inflammation through eating a diet rich in whole foods, organic, pasture-raised meats, and antioxidant rich foods
- Avoiding processed foods, consuming things in plastics, using artificial fragrances, consuming excessive alcohol and caffeine, and a sedentary lifestyle.
- Supplementation with magnesium, which is commonly depleted due to stress and a lack of it in our standard foods

Herbs and PCOS

Herbs known as allies for those with PCOS include vitex, spearmint, white peony root, licorice root, and cinnamon.

Many seek the medicine of **vitex** (*Vitex agnus-castus*) when hormonal imbalance related issues are present. But, as discussed in the section on general menstrual support, it's not that simple. Vitex usage could potentially be beneficial if used correctly in the right circumstances, or it can go awry. Vitex supports the body in producing progesterone and luteinizing hormones, which are essential for healthy, normal ovulation and balancing one's hormones, especially when estrogen dominance is present. Vitex will not work effectively if lifestyle changes do not shift as well. Like many herbs, it works slowly over a period of time. Typically, it must be used consistently for up to 3 to 6 months before noticeable changes occur. Often, folks find making better choices to support blood sugar and healthy inflammatory responses in conjunction with vitex renders the best results.

SAFETY NOTES: Vitex comes along with a laundry list of instances where it should not be used, which include depression, as it could worsen or inflict depressive episodes; when taking IVF drugs, as it can be too stimulating for the ovaries; and when taking hormonal birth control, as it could directly impact the effectiveness of it.

With this said, vitex may be an incredible short-term tool for PCOS through shifting the hormonal landscape by supporting ovulation. It is generally recommended as a tincture, but capsules may be effective as well.

Spearmint (*Mentha spicata*) is an herb applicable to those who experience elevated levels of testosterone, as it has been shown in studies to have an antiandrogen effect. A study done in 2007 showed that when participants drank spearmint tea 2 times a day for 5 days of the follicular phase, they showed a significant decrease in free testosterone and an increase in LH, FSH, and estradiol.[122] With this, I recommend using spearmint as a tea.

Ceylon cinnamon (*Cinnamomum verum*) is an herb regularly recommended for balancing blood sugar. And, with the

122 Mehmet Akdoğan, Mehmet Numan Tamer, Erkan Cüre, Medine Cumhur Cüre, Banu Kale Köroğlu, and Namik Delibaş, "Effect of Spearmint (Mentha Spicata Labiatae) Teas on Androgen Levels in Women With Hirsutism," *PTR. Phytotherapy Research/Phytotherapy Research* 21, no 5 (February 20, 2007): 444–47, doi.org/10.1002/ptr.2074.

high risk of insulin resistance with PCOS, this is an herb worth considering. Due to its ability to balance blood sugar, cinnamon may improve insulin resistance and has been shown in studies to assist in regulating the menstrual cycle of those with PCOS.[123] Research and anecdotal data shows that cinnamon may have an effect on oxidative stress and ovarian function.[124] It is often combined with **white peony root** (*Paeonia lactiflora*) for its ovarian tonic qualities, which also regulates ovarian function.[125] White peony reduces testosterone, increases low progesterone, and regulates estrogen and prolactin. Peony root also acts on the liver through anti-inflammatory actions and positive influences on gut microbiome.[126] This herb is also commonly paired with licorice root specifically in TCM and increasingly in western herbalism.

Licorice root (*Glycyrrhiza glabra*), on its own, is an adaptogenic adrenal fatigue tonic known for its use in regulating cortisol, which may promote the production of progesterone, thus assisting in cycle regulation. In tandem with peony, it has been shown to reduce testosterone levels and may alter LH and FSH. However, this combination is specific to a person and their current condition. It is paramount that you seek guidance from a practitioner to ensure it is the proper combination for you. This plant is also energetically and metaphysically balancing, offering sweetness and a synergistic quality to herbal tea blends and the body/mind.

123 "The Effect of Cinnamon on Polycystic Ovary Syndrome in a Mouse Model," *Reprod Biol Endocrinol*, (2015), rbej.biomedcentral.com/articles/10.1186/s12958-018-0418-y.

124 "Mechanistic and Therapeutic Insight into the Effects of Cinnamon in Polycystic Ovary Syndrome: A Systematic Review," (2019), ncbi.nlm.nih.gov/pmc/articles/PMC8502340/.

125 "Paeonia Lactiflora Improves Ovarian Function and Oocyte Quality in Aged Female Mice," *Animal Reproduction*, (2020), ncbi.nlm.nih.gov/pmc/articles/PMC7375873/.

126 "Menstrual Wellness and Menstrual Problems," In *Elsevier eBooks*, 97–185, 2010, doi.org/10.1016/b978-0-443-07277-2.00007-6.

OTHER SAFETY NOTES: Licorice root usage is not recommended for long-term use and should not be taken for longer than 2 weeks in a row. Those with heart failure, heart or liver or kidney disease, hormone-sensitive cancers, high blood pressure, low potassium, and diabetes should avoid the use of licorice root.

Herbs and Fibroids

Herbs used to support a body experiencing fibroids include black cohosh, lady's Mantle, and yarrow. Black cohosh is historically known to be a paramount herb for fibroids. However, due to habitat destruction and overharvesting in some areas, black cohosh is endangered in some areas and at-risk/threatened in others. For this reason, I do not recommend or teach extensively about black cohosh. This plant is mentioned here to serve as a reminder of the importance of ethical, sustainable harvesting practices. It is incredibly important to source herbs from farms and bulk herb sellers who have integrous harvesting and sourcing practices.

Lady's mantle (*Alchemilla vulgaris*) is not an herb I have used in excess with myself or with clients. None of this information is derived my personal, clinical experience but rather, information I have learned from books, research, and teachers over the years. Typically, I veer away from teaching about plants I have not intimately worked with, but this herb is one that comes up often when fibroids are discussed.I strongly felt it was worth mentioning here. Lady's mantle is anti-inflammatory in nature, with a specific affinity for toning the uterine muscles and lessening heavy bleeding. It is best described as an "ovarian regulator" which is "potently restorative," as Robin Rose Bennet states in her book, The Gift of Healing Herbs. It pairs well with raspberry leaf, and when needed, yarrow. I suggest using lady's mantle in the form of a tincture or tea.

Yarrow (*Alchemilla millefolium*) is an astringent, circulatory herb known for its warming, blood-purifying qualities. As fibroids are a cold, stagnant condition, yarrow's circulatory qualities have been used to clear out stagnant energy and blood that may be present in a uterus where fibroids are an issue. As yarrow can be drying, it may not be best used as a tonic. Formulation with other herbs that hold moistening qualities, such as chickweed, violet, marshmallow, or linden, should be considered.

Ginger root (*Zingiber officinale*) shares many similar qualities to yarrow, making it an effective remedy to use as a tonic when fibroids are present. Its anti-inflammatory and pain-relieving qualities are welcomed when painful menstruation is present. Its warming, dispersive nature works to break up thicker blood clots. Ginger may be effective for root cause issues related to digestion and elimination, as it quickens elimination and stokes the digestive fire, much like yarrow. All welcomed qualities for a body that needs to eliminate excess hormones and stress.

As Vitamin D deficiency is shown to be a risk factor for developing fibroids, Vitamin D supplementation should be considered.[127] If you are not receiving adequate sun exposure, consider taking a standard dosage of 2,000 IU a day. Ensure your Vitamin D supplement has a fat soluble element, as Vitamin D is made bioavailable with fat.

Herbs and Ovarian Cysts

In herbal medicine, cysts are viewed as stagnation in the lymph system, which is often why circulatory, lymph movers such as chickweed and calendula are often employed.

---

[127] "The Effect of Vitamin D Supplementation on the Size of Uterine Leiomyoma in Women with Vitamin D Deficiency," *Caspian Journal of Internal Medicine*, 2017.

Chickweed (*Stellaria media*) is known for cleansing the liver, moving stagnant fluids in the body, and providing deep nourishing minerals and vitamins to the body. It is cooling and moistening, a plant that shines in the first rains of spring. I've seen it clear persistent acne and psoriasis, as well as assist in dissolving ovarian cysts, which on an energetic level denotes its ability to clear heat and toxins from the body.

Calendula blossoms (*Calendula officinalis*) are a gentle lymphatic herb known for clearing fluid stagnation and curbing inflammation, which may be present with cysts. Calendula may be of assistance for healing after a cyst ruptures, specifically if it does so with extreme pain, as it is known as a wound healer, assisting blood movement and healing to a damaged area.

Both of these plants may be used in the form of herbal infusions or as tinctures.

From a holistic practices perspective, womb massage is specifically indicated here for its ability to bring movement to any stagnancy that is present. Consider making a salve or oil with any combination of rose, violet, mugwort, and ginger.

Herbs and Amenorrhea

Amenorrhea may exist for a wide variety of reasons, which means there is the possibility for many different root causes. For those who are amenorrheic for reasons other than hormonal birth control, some herbs that have been shown to assist in regulating the menstrual cycle include cinnamon and fennel.

High insulin levels[128] have been shown to have a strong tie to amenorrhea[129] and the hormones that regulate menstruation.

128 J. Niu, M. Lu, M., and B. Liu, :Association between Insulin Resistance and Abnormal Menstrual Cycle in Chinese Patients with Polycystic Ovary Syndrome," *Journal of Ovarian Research* 16, (2023), doi.org/10.1186/s13048-023-01122-4
129 "Correlation Between Menstruation Disorders and Insulin Resistance," (2003, June 1), *PubMed,* (June 1, 2003), pubmed.ncbi.nlm.nih.gov/14515662/

Due to its ability to improve insulin sensitivity,[130] **cinnamon** (*Cinnamomum verum*) may be a key ally for those with amenorrhea. Further, a random, controlled trial in 2014 showed that cinnamon improved menstrual cyclicity for those with PCOS.[131] While the type of cinnamon is not specified in many studies, I recommend using Ceylon cinnamon. Consider implementing cinnamon into your foods, as a tea, or tincture.

Fennel (*Foeniculum vulgare*) is a warming, spicy herb which has been used to support folliculogenesis[132] and acts as an emmenagogue to stimulate and increase menstrual blood flow. It has been shown to promote menstruation in those who experience amenorrhea with consistent use during the late follicular (once bleeding has ended), ovulatory, and luteal phases.[133] Fennel may be used culinarily, as a decoction, a capsule, or tincture.

Herbs and Miscarriage

After someone has endured a miscarriage, they undergo a healing process that spans beyond the physical. Like all types of pregnancy loss, one's mental, emotional, and spiritual space are affected when miscarriage occurs. For the physical body, it is paramount to rest, recover, and nourish one's body with whole,

130 B. Qin, K. S. Panickar, and R. A. Anderson "Cinnamon: Potential Role in the Prevention of Insulin Resistance, Metabolic Syndrome, and Type 2 Diabetes," *Journal of Diabetes Science and Technology*, 4 685–693, (2010), doi. org/10.1177/193229681000400324.

131 D. H. Kort and R. A. Lobo, R. A. "Preliminary Evidence that Cinnamon Improves Menstrual Cyclicity in Women with Polycystic Ovary Syndrome: A Randomized Controlled Trial, *American Journal of Obstetrics and Gynecology*, 211, (2014), 487. e1-487.e6. doi.org/10.1016/j.ajog.2014.05.009.

132 M. Khazaei, A. Montaseri, M. R. Khazaei, and M. Khanahmadi, (December 1, 2011), "Study of Foeniculum vulgare Effect on Folliculogenesis in Female Mice," PubMed Central (PMC). ncbi.nlm.nih.gov/pmc/articles/PMC4122825/.

133 F. Falahat, S. Ayatiafin, L. Jarahi, R. Mokaberinejad, H. Rakhshandeh, Z. Feyzabadi, and M. Tavakkoli, "Efficacy of a Herbal Formulation based on Foeniculum vulgare in Oligo/Amenorrhea: A Randomized Clinical Trial," *Current Drug Discovery Technologies* 17, 68–78, (2020), doi.org/10.2174/15701638156661 81029120512.

nourishing foods. Slow cooked meals. Slow movements. Resting as much as possible.

When blood loss happens, the use of **nettle leaf** (*Urtica dioica*) infusions is common as a supportive remedy. Its rich iron composition assists the body in building blood and nourishing the womb. It pairs well with **yarrow** (*Achillea millefolium*), which houses warming properties that circulate the blood and is incredibly healing to woundsites. **Raspberry leaf**, like nettle leaf, is a plant rich in minerals and vitamins known to assist in miscarriage recovery. Its toning and tightening properties are known to repair and restore health to the uterus more quickly. Consider pairing nettle and raspberry in an infusion and imbibing yarrow as a tincture or tea.

Cramp bark (*Viburnum opulus*) is a tool known for its use when threatened miscarriage is at stake. This plant works to cease uterine cramping and relax smooth muscle tissues. It is also useful in early labor as it may tone and regulate contractions, which can assist in a smoother delivery. If miscarriage does occur, cramp bark may be employed for its antispasmodic qualities, soothing cramps, and will effectively do so through a tincture or decoction.

Foods recommended during miscarriage, and all types of pregnancy loss, include seaweeds, which are rich in iron, iodine, calcium and other minerals and nutrients; warming, slow cooked foods which are easy to digest and bring much needed circulation to the body; porridges and oatmeals; bone broth, which offer bioavailable sources of collagen; foods which contain gelatin such as bone-in meats, homemade marshmallows, and homemade gummies; and dark, leafy greens.

For further support in pain management and in building the blood and health of the uterus, review the following information on herbs and abortion as the majority of the aftercare is similar.

Herbs and Abortion

There are many herbs that one can choose to use in preparation for, during, and after an abortion. Prior to an abortion, we look to use herbs that will tone and relax the uterus in preparation of the procedure or pill. After the abortion, we look to plants that will support the body through nausea, pain, anxiety, and blood building.

Red raspberry leaf (*Rubus idaeus*) has historically been used to prepare the uterus for abortion. As previously mentioned, this herb offers qualities that will relax, tone, and tighten the uterine muscles. Consider pairing raspberry leaf with **nettle leaf** (*Urtica dioica*), which, like raspberry leaf, is high in minerals and vitamins that will build the blood and assist the body in managing the changes it will be enduring during and after the abortion.

Herbs known for their capability to build the blood, support the liver, and cleanse the lymphatic system include dandelion and burdock root. If deep stress or nervous tension is present, chances are the body may need assistance with digestion. **Dandelion's** (*Taraxacum officinale*) cool, bitter qualities stimulate bile production, which assists in regulating and finessing digestion. It further cleanses the blood and supplies the body with antioxidants, minerals and vitamins such as vitamins K, A, and C, iron, calcium, magnesium, zinc, and others.

Burdock root (*Arctium lappa*) pairs well with dandelion root or can be used on its own. It is hepatoprotective, an herb that is thought to protect and rebuild the liver while also increasing the function of the liver. Like dandelion root, it has an impressive makeup, containing healthy prebiotic inulin, vitamin B-6, potassium, folate, and vitamin C.

SAFETY NOTE: If taking the abortion pill or on any other medications, please check with a healthcare provider before using these plants to ensure you are taking them within a timeframe that will not interact with the effectiveness of the pill or medications. A decoction of both of these roots is an effective way to receive their full spectrum of benefits. However, tinctures may be beneficial as well.

Cramping, low back pain, and abdominal pain may arise during and after the abortion. Herbs that may be useful for supporting the body at this time include California poppy, skullcap, and cramp Bark.

California poppy (*Eschscholzia californica*) is known as the opiate-less poppy, effective for its analgesic qualities and ability to calm the central nervous system, making it an effective ally when anxiety and tension is present. It is relaxing to the skeletal muscle system, is relaxing to blood vessels, and possibly improves blood flow. It is best used in a tincture and pairs well with skullcap, passionflower, and tulsi.

Skullcap (*Scuttellaria spp.*), like California poppy, is a nervine, historically used to rebuild a fried and overworked nervous system. I've used it for folks experiencing tension headaches and tight muscles, two things that may be present post-abortion. In my experience, it seemingly melts tightness away and opens a portal of relaxation. Use this plant as a tea or tincture.

Many people report feeling nauseated after taking the abortion pill. To quell these feelings, **ginger root** (*Zingiber officinale*) or **peppermint** (*Mentha piperita*) may be of assistance. As discussed, ginger is commonly used for morning sickness. Its affinity for effectively extinguishing nausea is applicable for a medley of issues related to nausea. When nervous tension, stress-induced digestive stress, or that "sick to my stomach" feeling arrives, consider reaching for ginger. This herb is commonly known for being calming to the digestive system, circulating to blood flow; and it may even help prevent vomiting. Use this plant as a decoction, syrup, tincture, or pastille.

Peppermint leaf may also be a soothing herbal ally when nausea and an upset stomach arrives. Its aromatic qualities are uplifting and opening to energetic blockages in the head. Menthol, the active constituent in peppermint, is antispasmodic and pain relieving, bringing in properties that are calming and soothing to digestive upset and discomfort. Tea, infused honey, or tincture are effective ways to imbibe the medicinal qualities of peppermint.

Herbs and Ectopic Pregnancy and C-Section

Ectopic pregnancy often requires surgery. And, a cesarean section is also a surgery. For these surgery-related experiences, we will focus on herbs known for their wound healing qualities such as rose hips and yarrow.

Rose hips (*Rosa spp.*) are an excellent bioavailable source of vitamin C, which assists in tissue repair and wound healing. Its antioxidant qualities combat free radical damage and oxidative stress, which likely improves the rate of wound healing.[134] Consider using this herbal medicine as a decoction, cold infusion, or jam. SAFETY NOTE: Do not use rose hips or Vitamin C supplements for 24 hours before surgery as it can reduce the effectiveness of anesthesia.

Yarrow (*Achillea millefolium*), the plant of one thousand flowers, is cooling and stimulating, bringing replenishing supplies of blood to areas which need it. It is known as an all-encompassing wound healer, effective at stopping a bleeding wound, bringing healing to wound sites, and assisting in new tissue growth. Pair it with raspberry leaf in a tea or tincture for more localized healing and strengthening to the uterine muscles.

---

134 "The Role of Antioxidants on Wound Healing: A Review of the Current Evidence," *Journal of Clinical Medicine*, ncbi.nlm.nih.gov/pmc/articles/PMC8397081/.

While baths are not indicated for those who have experienced abdominal surgery, consider creating a warm foot bath with powdered mustard seed, rosemary leaf, and ginger root, which will encourage warmth, circulation, and calming energies into the body.

Herbs and Molar Pregnancy

Review the herbs that were covered for abortion and ectopic pregnancy, for these may be applicable for a molar pregnancy depending on what symptoms are experienced and the treatments received for this type of pregnancy.

Herbs and Stillbirth

Herbs known for their nourishing qualities for a person that has endured a stillbirth may include nettle, raspberry leaf, yarrow, and St. John's Wort. **Nettle** (*Urtica dioica*) and **raspberry leaf** (*Rubus idaeus*), as we've discussed extensively in previous pages, are a dynamic duo which beholds a considerable amount of necessary minerals and vitamins needed for blood loss restoration, overall nourishment, and healing of the body. Raspberry leaf is a tool employed by countless midwives and doulas for postpartum healing of the uterine muscles, restoring tone and tightness to the area.

Yarrow (*Achillea millefolium*), as discussed for ectopic pregnancy, is a wholly effective plant for blood circulation, healing of wounds, and may assist in relieving pain after delivery. SAFETY NOTE: Please consult your healthcare provider before taking this herb as it interacts with some prescription medications and health conditions.

St. John's Wort (*Hypericum perforatum*), while known primarily for its antidepressant qualities, is effective for its wound healing properties. It is applicable for bruises and sore areas, which is why you may see it as an ingredient in herbal sitz baths for postpartum. SAFETY NOTES: SJW is extremely effective on the liver, so much so that it will knock most medications from the system before they have time to do the work they need to. For this, do not take SJW internally if taking any prescription drugs or supplements. However, topical use of SJW will not affect the effectiveness of medications. It may, however, create photosensitivity. If using SJW topically, avoid excessive sunlight.

Herbs for Tending to the Emotional Bodies

Pregnancy loss is generally a devastating and troubling time for those who were pregnant, as well as for their partners and families. This loss not only happens to the physical body, but touches us deeply in spiritual, mental, and emotional ways. For that, I have found plants offer a tremendous healing capacity, seemingly holding us in our heaviness in an ineffably tender way.

Many of these herbs are plants we have discussed throughout this book, which are also known to hold incredibly effective medicine for the emotional bodies during pregnancy loss. While they do not replace other therapies and practices that may bridge the healing process, they are a supportive addition to a holistic based approach. These therapies are recommended far beyond the scope of pregnancy loss and may be applied to anyone who feels called to use these plants.

Herbs for Anxiety and Stress

Tulsi, also known as Holy Basil (*Ocimum tenuiflorum*), is a nervine and adaptogen that simultaneously rebuilds and restores the nervous system while balancing the stress response. When anxiety and chronic stress occur excessively, the adrenals become enlarged and inflamed, sending out excessive amounts of cortisol. Tulsi has been shown in studies to curb this stress response, mitigating cortisol release and shrinking the adrenals back to their normal size.[135] Tulsi is calming, grounding, and soothing to tense, sad, and flustered energy.

Lemon Balm's (*Melissa officinalis*) sunny aromatics promote the clearing of one's mental space, gently relaxing while restoring the nervous system. It is antispasmodic, possibly assisting headaches and tummy aches associated with stress, tension, and worry. This plant pairs well with tulsi, rose, and passionflower.

Milky Oats (*Avena sativa*) is a sweet and cooling nourishing herb known well for its trophorestorative qualities through mending the fried and frayed myelin sheaths of our nerves through its nutritive properties, largely found in its milky sap. Milky oats tends to those who are chronically stressed, fatigued, and anxiety ridden. It is best used long-term, for its full range of qualities are not experienced until at least a month of use. Consider using it in tincture form, or as an infusion, steeped overnight.

When anxiety and stress feels so overwhelming that it feels as if your cup may run dry, I turn to **passionflower** (*Passiflora incarnata*). Passionflower is a nervine which is sedative, hypnotic, and relaxing, bringing qualities which may promote sleep, deep relaxation, and tension release. I typically do not recommend this herb for use during the day unless rest and relaxation are what is being promoted and needed. If cyclical, obsessive thought patterns are present, passionflower may be of assistance in stopping the hamster wheel. This plant pairs well with tonic usage of milky oats and rose, skullcap, tulsi, or lemon balm in the form of a tea or tincture.

---

135 M. Cohen, "Tulsi - Ocimum sanctum: A Herb for All Reasons," *Journal of Ayurveda and Integrative Medicine*, 5(4), 251, (2014), doi.org/10.4103/0975-9476.146554.

Ħerbs for Ġrief and Ħeartacħe

Motherwort (*Leonurus cardiaca*) tends to the heartspace. It is a physical and emotional cardiac tonic, working by way of its antioxidant and anti-inflammatory qualities to nurture the heart, and provides relief where tension is present. This plant hones in on its name, mothering those who are in need of TLC and support from their grief. It is calming to an overstimulated mind, and may promote the presence of joy when joy feels far from reach. As it is quite bitter, this plant is typically used as a tincture. And, if experiencing digestive issues, specifically due to the emotional landscape, may be used prior to meals to assist in assimilation of food and elimination.

Hawthorn's (*Crataegus spp.*) affinity for the heart runs deep. It is restorative to the entire cardiovascular system, strengthening capillaries and building up heart (and surrounding) tissues as well. It is no wonder that it has historically been used as an energetically protective heart plant for centuries. When one feels distanced from their heart, unable to process emotions, or unable to deal with grief, Hawthorne offers to hold these things through psycho-spiritual comfort. Hawthorn berry, leaf, or flower pairs well with rose and lemon balm. It may be taken in capsules, as an infusion, or in the form of a tincture.

SAFETY NOTE: Do note that Hawthorn should not be used with people who are taking blood pressure medications, along with many other medications. Please consult your healthcare provider before taking hawthorn.

Linden's (*Tilia*) "hug in a mug" qualities are ever welcomed to a body that has endured loss, trauma, and/or extended grief/heartache. Linden's leaves and blossoms are a relaxing nervine known for offering their uplifting, calming energetics. Where tension, irritability, sadness, loss for words, and heaviness lies, linden comes in to support.

Its gentle circulatory qualities may ease tensions, move stagnancy, and unwind cramps that are common symptoms of prolonged grief. This plant is a nourishing herb, meaning it may be steeped as an infusion for long periods of time to receive all of its medicinal qualities, especially when used as a tonic.

Aromatically, topically, and internally, **rose** (*Rosa spp.*) is a medicine that knows no bounds of attending to a heartspace stricken with grief. It is calming, protective, and literally works internally to strengthen the heart. When emotions are high, heat may be present in the body. Rose's cooling, astringent properties tighten up loose tissues and promote the literal healing of one's heart, which is incredibly important when deep heartache is involved. Rose pairs wonderfully with Linden, as they are both aromatic, cooling, and "heart hugging" energetically. Consider using it in a variety of ways, through hydrosol, infused honey, oxymel, or tincture.

Conclusion

*T*t is my prayer that the wisdom learned in these pages are insights helpful to your daily life, shared with those you love, and reflected upon for support throughout the cycles and stages we experience throughout our lives. Body literacy is a powerful and magickal resource. It is one that cannot be extracted. It is the torch of knowing, which cannot be destroyed as long as we are committed to offering its light to those that surround and come after us.

May you continue to use this book for inspiration on ways in which you can support your community and family through times of pregnancy loss or release, pregnancy and postpartum, puberty to menopause, and everything that exists in between. May you carry the nourishment instilled in these pages for the betterment of all wombs.

Before we part, I ask you to consider these questions as a meditation or a journaling session. May your answers invoke curiosity and reminders of what you've learned.

- What contained in this book has felt most impactful to you?
- What do you see differently now based off of something new you've learned?
- How does this impact other parts of your life?
- What surprised you most to learn?
- What do you feel a calling to implement in your own life?
- What herb do you wish to learn more about or work with?
- What medicines do you wish to create, whether with herbs or through ritual?

Make an offering to yourself in the form of a prayer, song, poem, dance, drawing, painting, or through any other act that affirms your dedication to the path of body literacy.

Herbal Glossary

Adaptogen - herbs which increase the body's response and resistance to stress

Alterative - herbs that work on the metabolic process to assist the body in the pathways of elimination, riding it of waste; also referred to as "blood cleansing" or "blood purifying"

Antispasmodic - herbs that relieve muscle spasms

Diuretic - herbs that assist in removing excess body fluid

Elixir - herbal medicine usually combining alcohol or vinegar and honey or maple syrup

Emmenagogue - an herb which stimulates or increases menstrual blood flow

Hepatic - herbs that tones, strengthens, and encourages the flow of bile in the liver

Galactagogue - herbs that increase or maintain breast milk production

Glycerite - herbal medicine made with herbs and glycerin as the main menstruum

Macerate - the soaking and steeping process during herbal medicine making

Menstruum - the solvent used in an herbal medicine

Mucilaginous - herbs which produce a viscous or gelatinous consistency

Nervine - herbs which support and calm the nervous system

Nootropic - enhances memory or other cognitive functions

Simples - the use of one herb at a time

Tincture - an herbal medicine which combines herbs and alcohol

Tonic - an herbal medicine which can be used over a long period of time to promote general well-being

Trophorestorative - herbs which have a restorative healing action on a specific organ or tissue

Appendix: Womb Resources

Pregnancy Loss and Release

- ectopic.org.uk
- abortionpillinfo.org
- consult.womenhelp.org
- plancpills.org
- reprocare.com
- mahotline.org
- abortioncarenetwork.org
- selfguidedabortion.com
- stillbirthday.com
- holisticabortions.com
- *You're The Only One I've Told: The Stories Behind Abortion* by Meera Sha
- *Creating Rituals for Pregnancy Loss*, zine by Red Door Collective

Reproductive Health and Education

- *Hormone Intelligence* by Aviva Romm
- *Taking Charge of Your Fertility* by Toni Weschler
- *The Fifth Vital Sign* by Lara Briden
- *Natural Birth Control Made Simple* by Hal C. Danzer and Barbara Kass-Annese
- *Let's Talk About Your Uterus: Body Conscious Birth Control* by Ashley Hartman Annis
- *Real Food for Pregnancy* by Lily Nichols
- *Real Food for Fertility* by Lily Nichols and Lisa Hendrickson-Jack

Reproductive Health Organizations

- marchofdimes.org
- postpartum.net

- guttmacher.org
- plannedparenthood.org

Teachers and Practitioners

- Taylor Jeffers, Clinical Herbalist and FEMM practitioner: lionheartedherbals.com
- Samantha Zipporah, Teacher and Author: samanthazipporah.com
- Lindsey Feldpausch (RH), Clinical Herbalist and Teacher: plantmatters.org
- Jim McDonald, Practitioner and Teacher: herbcraft.org
- Sage Mauer, Practitioner and Teacher, gaiaschoolofhealing.com
- The Herb Girls, Amy Wright and Eileen Schaeffer, Teachers and Practitioners: herbgirlsathens.com
- Samantha Phillips, Practitioner and Herbal Products: rootsofreverenceshop.com
- Erika Galentin (RH), Clinical Herbalist and Teacher: sovereigntyherbs.com

Food Blogs

- loveandlemons.com
- thedefineddish.com
- paleorunningmomma.com
- minimalisticbaker.com
- kalejunkie.com
- hummusapien.com
- oliviaadriance.com
- smittenkitchen.com
- ambitiouskitchen.com
- themediterraneandish.com

Herbalism

- *The Gift of Healing Herbs* by Robin Rose Bennet

- *Plant Spirit Medicine* by Eliot Cowan
- *Sacred Plant Medicine* by Stephen Harrod Buhner
- *The Witch's Herbal Apothecary* by Marysia Miernowska
- herbcraft.org
- *What a Plant Knows* by Daniel Chamovitz
- United Plant Savers
- *Wild Remedies* by Rosalee de la Forêt and Emily Han
- *The Encyclopedia of Herbal Medicine* by Andrew Chevallier
- *The Complete Book of Herbs* by Andi Clevely and Katherine Richmond
- *Principles and Practice of Phytotherapy* by Kerry Bone and Simon Mills
- *Herbal Materia Medica* by Michael Moore: free online resource: swsbm.com/ManualsMM/MatMed5.pdf
- *Braiding Sweetgrass* by Robin Wall Kimmerer
- *The Witch of the Forest's Guide to Earth Magick* by Lindsey Squire and Viki Lester

Herb Schools, Programs, and Apprenticeships

- The Gaia School of Healing
- Blue Otter School of Herbalism
- ArborVitae School of Traditional Herbalism
- Daoist Traditions College of Chinese Medical Arts
- Vermont Center for Integrative Herbalism
- Lindera: Jim McDonald's Energetic Folk Herbalism Program
- Chestnut School of Herbal Medicine
- The Herbal Academy
- Herbal Medicine for Women—Aviva Romm

Witchcraft

- *Inner Witch: A Modern Guide to the Ancient Craft* by Gabriella Herstik

- *Wild Witchcraft: Folk Herbalism, Garden Magic, and Foraging for Spells, Rituals, and Remedies* by Rebecca Beyer
- *The Green Witch* by Arin Murphy-Hiscock
- *The Cosmic Symposium: an Astrological Journey Through the Orchestra of the Planets* by Aubrey Houdeshell and Rose Ides
- *The Practical Witch's Almanac* by Friday Gladheart
- *Utopian Witch: Solarpunk Magick to Fight Climate Change and Save the World* by Justine Norton-Kerston
- *Disabled Witchcraft: 90 Rituals for Limited-Spoon Practitioners* by Kandi Zeller
- *Grimoire Girl: Creating an Inheritance of Magic and Mischief* by Hilarie Burton

Acknowledgments

The manuscript to this book sat in my computer for a year after its completion. I felt too nervous to pursue publishing—afraid that others would seek to misunderstand me through its material. While I have been "out of the broom closet" to my community for years, this louder proclamation felt scary in the day and age of social media where making a stance of who you are feels more vulnerable than before. Ultimately, I realized the information provided was more important than the fear I felt for the judgment of identifying as a witch and continued onwards toward finding a home for my book.

A book does not come together without the assistance and aid of a wide-reaching community. With that, I want to thank Microcosm Publishing for seeing the worth in Womb Witch and choosing to publish this book, among the many other great titles and authors they represent. Thank you to Kandi Zeller, my editor, whose insights, ideas, and edits were invaluable to making this book into what it is now.

As I wrote, edited, and expanded this book, I sought the stories, advice, and expertise of my community. To those that shared their stories of birth, menstruation, and other womb experiences, as well as the knowledge that allowed for this book to feel inclusive and wholly holistic, I am forever grateful. Truly.

I thank my clients, Julez Waldeck, Brooke Bednarz, Hannah Bates, my Aunt Janey Kevan, Aubrey Houdeshell, Hannah Clemons, Edgar Cisneros, Stewart Brahler, Bailey McAvenia, Kelly Phillips, Kartika Klaresta, Mary Maley, Savannah LeCornu, Kai Wolfe, Jessica Vellela, Jason Baldwin, Vivienne Gerard, Alison Bartish, Madeline Cisneros, Sophia Pardini, Britany Pope, Jeana Anderson, and Keriann Uno —all people who had heartfelt and meaningful conversations with me about my writing process, what I was writing and who I was writing it for.

To Leslie Keating, who helped remind me that the path of the witch was not one to fear, but to behold. May your spirit live on in these pages.

To Kelli Williams, a bright star in my life, your strength, wisdom, and fierce love in telling yours, Chris's, and Noah's story is one I know changes lives and allows others to feel seen—I am so proud of the woman and mother you are.

To Taylor Jeffers: your insights and knowledge-base surrounding fertility awareness and education as a clinical herbalist were instrumental in adding necessary points in this book. Thank you so, so, so much.

To Sara Totri, without whom this book would have seriously struggled to come together. Thank you for the gift of a spare laptop when mine decided to turn into a black screen. And thank you for your friendship, support, and encouragement when I was in the early stages of turning this manuscript into a book; it meant more than you know.

I want to thank my Mom, Dad, and siblings, Becca and Brian, for their support as a whole. For as long as I can remember, I've claimed that one day I will publish a book. And, when I came to tell them this would be the book I was going to publish first, they could not have been more supportive, proud, and encouraging. Thank you to my sweet sister and best friend, Becca, for your thoughtful edits, always cheering me on from the sidelines, and understanding me in ways that only a sister could.

To my partner Dave, thank you for holding a grounded, loving space for me that feels freeing, expansive, and safe all at once. Writing this book was no easy feat, and over the years I wrote and worked on this project, you were supportive during every step. I am constantly in awe of your willingness to dream big with me and truly show up as my partner and best friend. I am forever grateful that you have graced my life.

To my Grandma Merritt, who passed away as I was completing this book and asked about my book writing process every step of the way. You were one of the greats of my life and believed in me in such a sincere, loving way. What an honor it was to be your granddaughter. Thank you for teaching me to be fierce and kind at the same time; that creating a meal or a sweet treat for someone is a beautiful pathway to showing love in a physical form; and that love expressed through warmth and without judgment beholds strength, truth, and wholeness. I love you. I will forever miss you. Until we meet again.

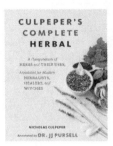
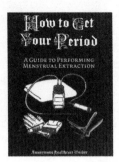
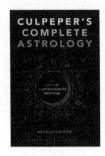

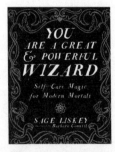
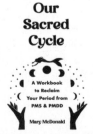
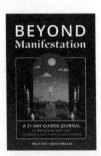

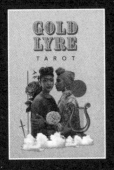

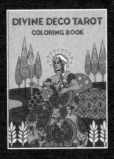

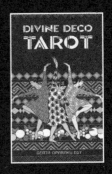

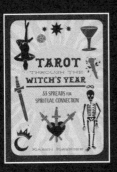

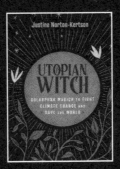

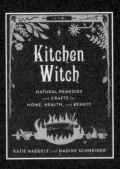

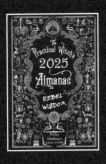

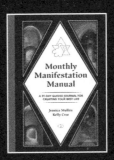

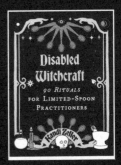

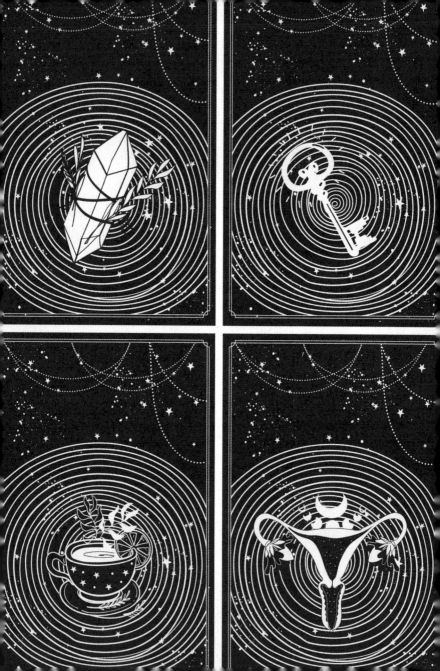

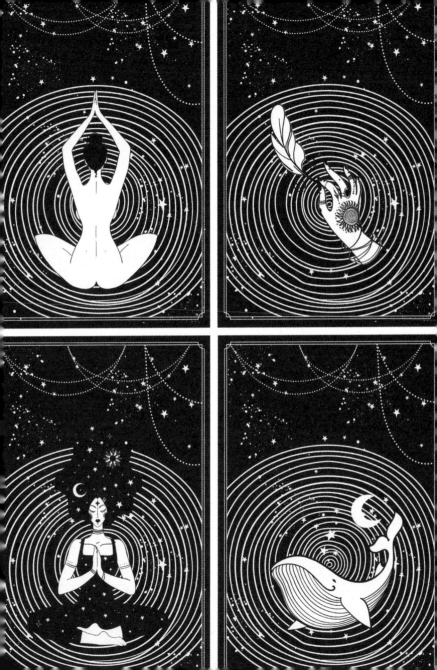

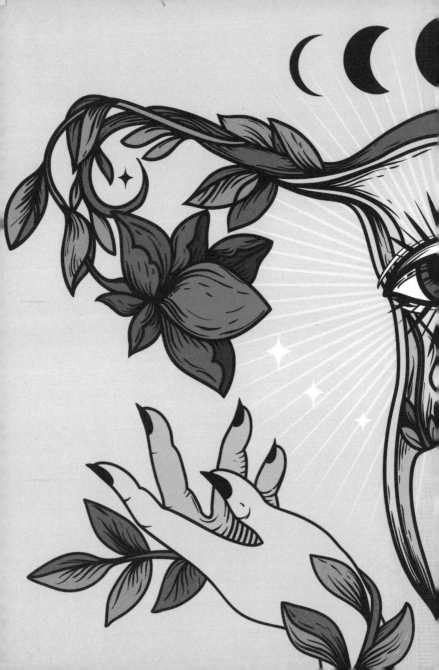